A Doctor's Guide to Essential Rewards

12 Months to Clean Living

Olivier Wenker, MD, DEAA, ABAARM, MBA

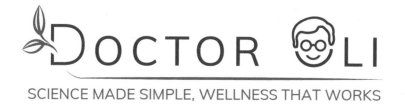

DOCTOR OLI

SCIENCE MADE SIMPLE, WELLNESS THAT WORKS

ISBN# 978-0-9600065-0-2

Printed in the United States of America

Visit doctoroli.com to purchase additional copies.

For information about speaking engagements or to host a book signing, contact team@doctoroli.com with "Events" in the subject line.

Edited by Dana Schorr and Megan Wenker

Content Edited by Ellen Wenker, Lic Phil I

Photo Credit: Samuel Schorr, Ph.D.

Table of Contents

Dedication

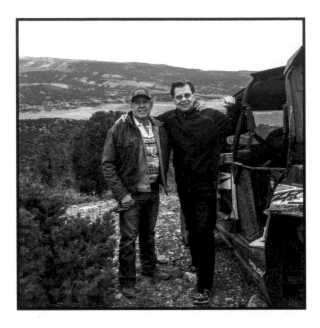

This book is dedicated to D. Gary Young, the well-known pioneer in essential oils, whose vision of bringing healthy products into every home inspired me to write this.

Gary was not just a visionary, but also a truly wonderful human being and the greatest and most loyal friend I ever had. My whole aim is to spread his message of health to all mankind and to help everyone move forward in the spirit of Gary.

Foreword

Really? Doctor Oli is writing a book about Essential Rewards? I was immediately curious and wanted to see what he had to say. I was so surprised. After I read the first few pages, I was captivated and wanted to read more.

No one has written a book like this before, especially from his medical viewpoint. He gives a lot of information for those who want it, with voluminous documentation for the skeptic who wants proof. For those who just want to know which products to order each month, there is a simple explanation of the target group for any given month.

This is perfect for new members who are wondering how to start with a good program that takes them through an entire year. Not only are they ordering a variety of products, but they are also becoming educated about different product categories. Even those who have been members for a while and are quite familiar with the products might discover that they have been missing something or that they like the organized way the program changes from month to month.

We all know that the Essential Rewards Program is an important key to building a business and maintaining member activity and interest. The benefits are amazing, but each member needs the education in order to be motivated. Doctor Oli's book is very informative, helpful, and caring, with clever titles and fun pictures. Members who read it will benefit in their own individual way.

Thanks, Doc, for helping members to not only get started but to also keeping them going as they Journey On, living with passion while fulfilling their dreams.

-**Mary Young**, CEO of Young Living Essential Oils

Making the Change

ᒿCHAPTER 1

My Why

Writing this book and getting it into the hands of many people is so important to me, thanks to a crazy event in my life. Several years ago, I was diagnosed with a very rare disease called Miller-Fisher Syndrome. This is a subtype of the better-known Guillain-Barré Syndrome, where antibodies start destroying myelin nerve sheaths of mostly peripheral nerves.

With Miller-Fisher Syndrome, this damage is basically isolated to the brain, including the nerves leaving the brain. Both are neurological conditions that cause mild to severe muscle weakness. The damage to the brain and nerves is triggered by an immune system reaction against certain proteins in the tissue that are important for movement, sensation, and function.

The human body confuses the proteins in the brain tissue or nerve sheaths with bacterial or viral proteins, leading to an antibody response with subsequent brain and nerve damage.[1] The typical symptoms of this rare condition are complete ataxia (the loss of full control of bodily movements), eye problems, and lack of deep tendon nerve reflexes.[2]

According to the National Ataxia Foundation, common symptoms of ataxia are a lack of coordination, slurred speech, trouble eating and swallowing, eye movement abnormalities, deterioration of fine motor skills, difficulty walking, gait abnormalities, tremors, and heart problems.[3]

Individuals with ataxia often require the use of wheelchairs, walkers, and/or scooters to aid in their mobility. Eye problems, also called ophthalmoplegia, cause double vision, blurred sight, disorientation, and dizziness. The problems can come from damage in the little nerve sheaths of the eye muscles and/or from damage of the eye coordination point in the brain stem.

Since I typically always go all the way, it was no different with this disease. Of course, I had to get an extreme form of it, leaving me severely handicapped. Since I had just spent a week in the Caribbean, the medical specialty teams suspected a Zika virus infection as the culprit of my Miller-Fisher Syndrome. However, at that time there was no test yet for Zika virus antibodies.

So, long story short, after leaving the hospital in a wheelchair, expecting not to walk for a long time, or maybe with a walker for the rest of my life, everything suddenly changed. I was especially devastated because in just a few months, I was supposed to walk my only daughter down the aisle.

Since I had exhausted all possible treatment options of modern medicine, I started to search for alternative means to support my recovery. I called my friend Gary Young, internationally known for his expertise in using plant-based remedies and essential oils, and asked him for advice.

Combining our experiences led to a health-supporting protocol for me. It became very important to stop any further damage to my nervous system, wherever that damage might come from.

At that time, I had been a speaker for Young Living for several years, and my family and I knew about the importance of products free of harsh chemicals. Toxins and heavy metals, including those found in food and beverages, personal care products, household products, and the environment, are known to accumulate in fatty tissue of humans.

The brain and the nerves are highly fatty organs. Therefore, any exposure to herbicides, pesticides, toxins, or heavy metals would further attack my brain in addition to messing up my hormone balance and overall health.

I started to intensely study the medical literature to see what I could do to avoid these bad chemicals. As a physician, I had already seen firsthand what the increased toxic burden in our world did to my patients, like heavy occurrence of disease, unbalanced hormone levels, and decreased fitness and wellness. Harsh chemicals are even called endocrine disruptors, because they profoundly change our hormone balance which then leads to a variety of problems.

I had to make major adjustments to my own life. My wife Ellen and I completely overhauled our lifestyles and made sure to replace every remaining toxic product used in our home with Young Living's healthy alternatives. I survived my illness and walked my daughter down the aisle. I am now fully recovered from my medical condition.

This outcome astonished me, and sharing this information suddenly became very personal. I made it my mission to inform and educate others about the importance of avoiding harsh chemicals while promoting a healthy, active lifestyle.

I started to learn more about history, nature, and alternative medicines so that I could stand on stage and teach others. And the more I was researching, reading, understanding, and discussing these findings with Gary Young, the more I knew that I needed to share the same message he had been carrying around the world for decades.

Gary, living in the world of integrative and alternative, natural plant-based methods, and I, living in the modern world of medicine full of pharmaceutical drugs and prescriptions, met somewhere in the middle. We believed that enjoying the technology of modern diagnostics and personalized medicine while incorporating the plant-based, natural ways God had entrusted us with was the best compromise.

So, I became a "BioHacker." A BioHacker changes the outcome of disease to one of wellness by influencing proteins in the body that attach to the DNA and define how certain genes are expressed. This field is also called "Epigenetics." It is important to know that positive and negative changes can be inherited and therefore influence the health of generations to come.

Still not convinced? Well, read on to find out for yourself what we humans have been doing to ourselves over the past few decades, and what changes we caused not only in our own health but also in the environment.

Endocrine Disruptors: The Silent Killers

According to the Environmental Working Group Cosmetics Database, an average person in the United States uses nine personal care products each day, containing a total of 126 unique chemical ingredients. More than 25% of all women, and one out of every 100 men, use at least 15 personal care products daily.[4]

This is not only an issue in the United States, either. A research poll by a cosmetic company showed that women in the United Kingdom are exposed to 515 toxic and harsh chemicals every day.[5] So far I am only talking about your basics, like shampoo, conditioner, deodorant, lotion, cream, cologne or perfume, and cosmetics. Most of these are applied before breakfast.

Those high numbers do not even include all the toxins and endocrine-disrupting (hormone-changing) chemicals used in common household products, air fresheners, laundry detergents, dryer sheets, soaps, candles, and other similar products.

A study spearheaded by the Environmental Working Group (EWG) detected 287 chemicals in the umbilical cord blood of newborns, 180 of which are known to cause cancer in humans or animals, 217 of which are toxic to the brain and nervous system, and 208 of which cause birth defects or abnormal development in animal tests. On average, a baby had 200 industrial chemicals and pollutants in its umbilical cord blood.[6]

Toxins and harsh chemicals are known to be endocrine disruptors, which means that they change the type and levels of hormones in our body. In fact, chemicals are also called "xeno-estrogens." "Xeno," from ancient Greek, means "foreign or from the outside," and estrogens are the main female hormones. Xeno-estrogens absorb into the body, attach to estrogen receptor sites, and change the way your body works.

Several studies looked at the effects of pesticides, herbicides, and fertilizers in the waterways and found an almost complete lack of male fish. Almost 100% of the fish has been feminized by these endocrine disruptors. Over 90% of the male fish had eggs in their testicles and were labelled "intersex" fish.[7] Sperm production and quality in these male intersex fish were severely impaired.[8]

Other studies looked at frogs and found that herbicide endocrine disruptors caused complete feminization and chemical castration in the males.[9] As a result, one in ten male frogs became a fully functioning female, and 75% of the male frogs had no more sperm nor testosterone and could not reproduce anymore.

These endocrine disruptors are disastrously affecting the environment. We humans are causing this destruction but completely underestimate the impacts of these chemicals.[10] And it is not just animals that suffer these consequences.

A huge body of medical literature describes the negative effects of xeno-estrogenic chemicals on male and female reproductive health. Over the past few decades, we have seen a steady decline in human fertility.[11] More couples struggle to have children than ever before, and when they do finally procreate, they pass on genetically changed information to their offspring.

A growing number of human studies, conducted in the last 10 years, describe obesogenic (fat inducing) chemicals as being important cofactors in the increasing rate of obesity around the world.[12] The effects of exposure to these estrogenic chemicals are crucially important during developmental phases of life, when pre-programming for an adipogenic outcome (the future body weight of a person) may occur.

These obesogenic toxins and chemicals might also predispose individuals to gain weight despite their efforts to limit caloric intake and increase levels of physical activity.[13]

Because most toxins and chemicals are stored in fatty tissue, there seems to be a vicious cycle: the more toxins and chemicals absorb into the body, the higher the chance for increased fat mass (obesity). And the higher the number and size of fat cells, the more toxins and chemicals can be stored, hence increasing the risk for obesity again.

The global health and economic burden related to toxic environmental chemicals is in excess of millions of deaths and billions of dollars every year.[14] It involves all aspects of human and animal life: changing hormones, increased infertility, higher risk of obesity, cardiovascular disease, neurological and developmental problems, changes in the bacterial composition of the microbiome in the gut and on the skin, cancers, and plenty of other health-related issues.

There is also increasing evidence that these toxins and chemicals not only affect your own body and health, but that they also affect your children and grandchildren via transgenerational impacts caused by epigenetic changes.

Endocrine disrupting chemicals can change the human epigenome.[15] The epigenome is defined as a collection of proteins and other compounds that can attach to the DNA and therefore modify the way genetic information is expressed. Your offspring can then inherit these changes. Your choices today will impact future generations.

Make Your Change

It's time for all of us to rethink what we're doing. Are you ready to make a difference for yourself, your family, your pets, and your home? Are you ready to make a difference for your local environment, for others, for our future generations, and for Mother Earth?

If your answer is **YES**, keep reading to learn the easy ways in which you can make a difference. I will guide you through a system which will refresh your life, your environment, your energy, and your overall health and wellness, all while having the opportunity to save you money.

There are many ways to make personal changes and create a difference in this world. There is a good chance, that by the time you read this, someone has already approached you to become part of an international movement started by Gary Young almost three decades ago.

He founded Young Living Essential Oils, an amazing company that provides more than 500 healthy products for you to easily make smart decisions that will have a major impact on you, your family, and the world. By using these products, which are formulated without any toxins but are full of health-promoting compounds, not only will you avoid further accumulation of toxins and endocrine-disrupting chemicals in your body, but you will also decrease the negative impact these chemicals have on the environment and Mother Earth.

Why would I as a physician be interested in the Essential Rewards program of Young Living Essential Oils? The answer is simple; because it's a great opportunity to help yourself build a healthy lifestyle, save money, get the best deal, and enjoy financial stability. Worrying about money is a big contributor to stress which negatively impacts all aspects of overall health and social wellbeing.

I believe the Essential Rewards program will benefit everyone. To make it easy for you, I will share my thoughts from a scientific perspective on how to support your quest for all around wellness.

As a physician, I ask you to consult with your own healthcare provider before taking, applying, smelling, or otherwise consuming any Young Living products, especially if you are taking any medications or suffer from any health conditions.

The rules and guidelines in the United States allow us to make "Structure/Function Claims" when talking about products registered with the FDA as nutritional supplements. The FDA website defines these claims as the following:

> Structure/function claims may describe the role of a nutrient or dietary ingredient intended to affect the normal structure or function of the human body, for example, "calcium builds strong bones." In addition, they may characterize the means by which a nutrient or dietary ingredient acts to maintain such structure or function, for example, "fiber maintains bowel regularity," or "antioxidants maintain cell integrity."[16]

Young Living has labelled several essential oils as dietary supplements (in the U.S. we call this the Vitality line). Therefore, one would be able to cite some scientific findings when talking or writing about these oils. However, the source should always be listed and the content of the scientific papers should be cited correctly. For this reason, I added the citations and references of the scientific papers I used to write this book.

You should also know that basically all scientific studies about essential oils use synthetic essential oils, or only individual components of essential oils. Since Young Living only sells pure essential oils, it is unlikely that their products are used for scientific research studies. Researchers hate when the components of a natural substance vary according to location, climate, and other variables. That makes it much more difficult to obtain clear research results. To my knowledge, none of the studies cited in this book used Young Living Essential Oils for their research. Therefore, we cannot automatically deduce that the same study result could be obtained when using a Young Living Essential Oil or oil blend.

Most statements regarding household or cleaning products are regulated by the Environmental Protection Agency (EPA). It is important to realize that when talking about Young Living household products, we should use the term "formulated without toxins" and not "free of any toxins or toxic chemicals."

You will also see that this book is very well researched. To enable you to come to your own conclusions, I have added all of the references I used for writing this book. You'll find almost 600 citations. Since this is a book and not a scientific paper, I decided to use an abbreviated form of citations in order to make it more readable for non-scientists. For simplicity, I decided not to list the names of the authors. So I would like to thank all of the authors for their contributions to science and medicine.

References:

[1] Miller Fisher Syndrome. StatPearls Publishing; 2018.

[2] Miller Fisher's syndrome. Semin Neurol. 2012 Nov;32(5):512-6. doi: 10.1055/s-0033-1334470.

[3] National Ataxia Foundation. What Is Ataxia? https://ataxia.org/what-is-ataxia/.

[4] Exposures add up – Survey results. Environmental Working Group Cosmetics Database. http://www.ewg.org/skindeep/2004/06/15/exposures-add-up-survey-results/#.W3cvguhKiUl.

[5] https://www.reuters.com/article/us-britain-cosmetics/average-uk-woman-wears-515-chemicals-a-day-idUSTRE5AI3M820091119.

[6] The Pollution in Newborns: A Benchmark Investigation Of Industrial Chemicals, Pollutants And Pesticides In Umbilical Cord Blood https://www.ewg.org/research/body-burden-pollution-newborns#.W3heWehKiUk.

[7] Intersex (testicular oocytes) in smallmouth bass from the Potomac River and selected nearby drainages. J Aquat Anim Health. 2007 Dec;19(4):242-53. doi: 10.1577/H07-031.1.

[8] Reproductive endocrine disruption in smallmouth bass (Micropterus dolomieu) in the Potomac River basin: spatial and temporal comparisons of biological effects. Environ Monit Assess. 2012 Jul;184(7):4309-34. doi: 10.1007/s10661-011-2266-5.

[9] Atrazine induces complete feminization and chemical castration in male African clawed frogs (Xenopus laevis). Proc Natl Acad Sci U S A. 2010 Mar 9; 107(10): 4612–4617. doi: 10.1073/pnas.0909519107.

[10] Pesticide mixtures, endocrine disruption, and amphibian declines: are we underestimating the impact? Environ Health Perspect. 2006 Apr;114 Suppl 1:40-50.

[11] Human infertility: are endocrine disruptors to blame? Endocr Connect. 2013 Sep 1; 2(3): R15–R29. doi: 10.1530/EC-13-0036.

[12] Role of Environmental Chemicals in Obesity: A Systematic Review on the Current Evidence. J Environ Public Health. 2013; 2013: Article ID 896789. doi: 10.1155/2013/896789.

[13] Endocrine disruptors and obesity. Nat Rev Endocrinol. 2015 Nov;11(11):653-61. doi: 10.1038/nrendo.2015.163.

[14] International Federation of Gynecology and Obstetrics opinion on reproductive health impacts of exposure to toxic environmental chemicals, Int J Gynecol Obstet (2015), http://dx.doi.org/10.1016/j.ijgo.2015.09.002.

[15] Multigenerational and transgenerational effects of endocrine disrupting chemicals: A role for altered epigenetic regulation? Semin Cell Dev Biol. 2015 Jul;43:66-75. doi: 10.1016/j.semcdb.2015.05.008.

[16] U.S. Food and Drug Administration FDA. Structure/Function Claims. https://www.fda.gov/Food/LabelingNutrition/ucm2006881.htm.

✌CHAPTER 2

Essential Rewards: Clean Living Delivered to Your Doorstep

Because this is not just a one-time effort, smart choices need to be made on a regular, if not daily, basis, and not just sometimes. Those who walk this path will continually experience positive results. The best way to make these changes, and stick to them, is to enroll in Young Living's highly valuable and advantageous Essential Rewards (ER) subscription program, which will save you substantial amounts of money while accomplishing your new wellness goals.

I made it easy for you to make these changes with this year-long product ordering guide. In my opinion as a healthcare professional, the first six months are absolutely critical, especially for newcomers. The following six months contain suggestions for more specialized interests, such as "Work It Out" for anyone who wants to adopt a more active lifestyle, or "Baby Talk" for anyone with a baby or small child in their life. These latter months can be rearranged as desired, depending on your family's needs You can always repeat any months that have your "must-have" products.

So, my message to you is loud and clear. Change your life, the lives of your loved ones and pets, and the poor state of the environment. Commit to it. Go all the way. Don't be afraid. Change your habits by improving your lifestyle and buying cleaner, safer products.

We cannot make a significant change by using healthy products occasionally. We need to use them every day, in our home, on our bodies, everywhere. If we do, not only will we improve our health, but we can contribute to saving Mother Earth.

Imagine the difference we can all make if we choose to use better products and to make better lifestyle decisions, month after month. It was Gary's dream, and now it is my dream as well. This is why I wrote this book, *A Doctor's Guide to Essential Rewards*. Gift it to your new team members so that they not only have an easy, beautiful guideline on WHAT to order every month, but also the WHY. This guide is also available as a mini version for affordable, easy sharing with your friends and team members. The mini is the step-by-step monthly ordering guide with much less science.

While this book is focused on changing out the daily products you use on your body and in your home, I would certainly add more essential oils. So, I included a "Bonus Oil" suggestion to fit with each monthly theme, for those of you who want to beef up your essential oil collection which was started when you purchased your Premium Starter Kit.

As a father, I know how important it is to have happy, healthy children. In addition to the Bonus Oil each month, I also included a KidScents® product recommendation. Your kids can join you on the path to cleaner living and enjoy the Young Living options formulated just for them.

The Essential Rewards Subscription Program

These days, you can subscribe to receive a box of anything, from healthy groceries with recipes, to clothing, and even books. Amazon even offers a five percent discount on their "subscribe and save" order method.

Young Living takes the monthly ordering concept to a whole new level with their Essential Rewards program. Wholesale members receive 24% off the retail price and earn a percentage of their purchase back in points to be used toward future Quick Orders.

In addition, members receive free monthly promo products based on order volume and free gifts for membership anniversaries. Does this sound too good to be true? Even better, YOU get to choose the products to receive each month. Try something new or restock your favorites, it's up to you. There is no purchase obligation, so you can cancel at any time. In fact, Young Living has taken the Essential Rewards program a step further and now offers a priority shipping program similar to Amazon Prime.

So, I've based my whole book around cleaning up your household and lifestyle by using Young Living products purchased through Essential Rewards. Your Premium Starter Kit (PSK) can be your first Essential Rewards order. This is amazing because you will automatically earn $10 back from the purchase of the PSK. For the sake of ease and clarity, in my writings I assume your first month on ER is my Month 1 order suggestion.

Essential Rewards Points

Earn points toward future purchases with every Essential Rewards order. As your months of ordering with Essential Rewards increase, so do your rewards. In the first 3 months of consecutive Essential Rewards membership, you receive

10% of your overall Essential Rewards purchases back as credits. From months 4 to 24, you will receive 20% back, and when you are on the program for more than 24 consecutive months you will earn 25% of your purchases back as credits. You can use these credits towards getting products for free.

Essential Rewards Loyalty Gifts

Earn gifts available only to members of the Essential Rewards program when you place consecutive Essential Rewards orders over 50 PV. Point Value (PV) is the total value of your purchase, in points, independent of any currency. Enjoy your rewards when you consecutively order for the first three, six, and nine months. You will also receive the exclusive Loyalty™ Essential Oil blend after your 12th consecutive month and every 12 months thereafter.

Exclusive Bonus Products

Every month, if you order a certain amount (usually 100, 190, 250, and 300 PV in the US), you receive free "promo" products. The higher the purchase amount, the more free products that stack up. If you are placing these orders via Essential Rewards, you receive an additional exclusive product.

Easy Monthly Shipments

Enjoy the convenience of automatic monthly shipments. Just set up your order and kick back as all of your favorite products are sent right to your doorstep month after month. So, after you've followed my guide for six to twelve months, you can easily add your "Must Have" products to your order that automatically arrives at your doorstep each month.

Discounted Shipping

Essential Rewards orders qualify for discounted shipping rates. Reduced price shipping options vary based on weight and shipping method.

YL Go and YL Go+

Enrolling in Essential Rewards also unlocks access to YL Go and YL Go+, the exclusive shipping subscription options that offer fast, easy, and free shipping with priority processing.

These are programs similar to Amazon Prime. By paying an annual subscription fee, you get several advantages. YL Go offers 13 free shipments per year and YL Go+ offers 25 free shipments per year. Both plans offer an affordable flat rate overnight shipping option.

If you are on Essential Rewards, you need to be on YL Go, which gives you 12 monthly shipments and at least one order with rewards points in a year. It will certainly save you money on shipping over the next year, and you will receive your products faster.

Eligibility for Commission/Check Issuance

With the minimum requirement of 100PV, you become eligible to receive a commission check and have the peace of mind that your required amount of PV is generated automatically.

Many of Young Living's top leaders started their Young Living business purely to be able to buy their oils and products for free. Most never thought they would retire from their 9-to-5 jobs, and have a life of financial freedom, just by sharing Gary's mission to get Young Living Essential Oils into every household. (View Young Living's income disclosure statement at youngliving.com/ids.)

My monthly order suggestions in this guide are always at 100PV or more. If you are unable to commit 100PV per month to your healthy lifestyle mission, at least order the 50PV Essential Rewards minimum. You will still reap the benefits, but it will take you twice as long to fully enjoy a clean lifestyle.

Not every month evenly splits into two orders of 50PV. Therefore, some months may require you to add additional products. I suggest you add the Bonus Oil at the end of each chapter if you need to get to 50 PV.

The Importance of the Essential Rewards Program

An analysis of the organization of a Royal Crown Diamond, the highest leadership rank achievable in Young Living, revealed that after 15 months, only two percent of people who signed up with a Premium Starter Kit, but did not enroll in Essential Rewards, continued to order products monthly. However, basically 100% of people who signed up with a Premium Starter Kit plus an ER subscription were still ordering 15 months later.

Another internal analysis of a Crown Diamond's organization revealed that in any given month almost 90% of members with orders were in fact members on ER.

Between the credits, bonuses, free products, reduced shipping, and other benefits, the monetary savings are substantial and add up quickly. There is no better way to live clean and make a difference in the world than by signing up for Young Living's Essential Rewards subscription program.

Get Started

First, make sure you are enrolled as a Young Living Wholesale Member before you sign up for Essential Rewards. Check in with the person who gave you this book to get their member number, so you can list them as your referral source and get on their team.

If and ONLY if, you found this book on your own and you are not yet a Young Living Member, send an email to team@doctoroli.com. We will be happy to guide you in your healthy lifestyle journey.

Second, add the Month 1 products from this guide as your first Essential Rewards order by typing in the item number found in this book. Young Living has a multitude of great products. If you need to find an alternative due to market availability, you have many options. For example, Cool Azul Sports Gel can be a good substitute for Cool Azul Pain Cream.

Third, set up PV Assistant. Since all of our essential oils are 100% pure, the volume of oil distilled is often dependent on weather conditions, which affect crop yields. Seasonal conditions can cause variance in product availability. Therefore, items may go out of stock making it difficult to fulfill a specific product in your monthly Essential Rewards order.

When that happens, the total monthly amount spent is reduced and can possibly fall below the 100 PV required to be eligible for a commission check, or the 50 PV required for ER orders to process. With PV Assistant, you can create a monthly PV goal, as well as a wish list of your favorite Young Living products.

If your Essential Rewards order ever falls below your customizable PV goal, the PV Assistant will automatically add an item from your wish list so that you always meet your goal. Everyone on Essential Rewards should have the PV Assistant.

To manage or change your monthly Essential Rewards order, simply log in to your Virtual Office (https://www. youngliving.com/vo/#/login) and make the appropriate changes or contact Member Services (1-800-371-3515) who will assist you with a live operator.

Most of this information and text describing the Essential Rewards subscription program is directly from Young Living Essential Oils, LC, and can be found online at youngliving.com

KidScents® and Loyalty™ are trademarks of Young Living Essential Oils, LC.

CHAPTER 3

Fire Up Your Engines with NINGXIA RED®

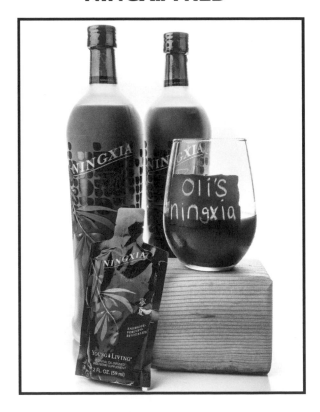

Oxygen is indispensable for life. When cells use oxygen, free radicals are created as a consequence of energy production in the mitochondria. Free radicals can also be created as a result of overall stress, radiation, increased metabolism, bad nutrition, disease, and pollution. Their accumulation in the body generates a phenomenon called oxidative stress.

A little oxidative stress might be okay, but when it becomes overwhelming, the results can be negative. Too much oxidative stress is known to be a factor in the etiology (cause) of several chronic and degenerative diseases.[17,18] Cell membranes are particularly rich in unsaturated fatty acids and are sensitive to oxidation reactions.[19] The DNA at the core of the cells carrying our genetic information is the target of severe attacks by these free radicals.

Fortunately, there are steps you can take with your nutrition to offset some of these effects. The plant Lycium barbarum produces a fruit which is also known as wolfberry, goji or gogi berry, or gouqizi. It is also known as the Ningxia wolfberry because it grows in the Ningxia region of Northern China. It is one of the most widely used and scientifically studied plants in Chinese herbal medicine. The Ningxia wolfberry helps the body eliminate free radicals effectively and enhances the activity of antioxidant enzymes. One scientific review concluded that Ningxia wolfberry intake produces an almost 10% increase in serum antioxidant capacities in human subjects under normal conditions.[20] It also activates other endogenous antioxidants that are produced by your body, thereby multiplying the free radical scavenging in the different organ systems.[21]

Ningxia wolfberries contain abundant Lycium barbarum polysaccharides (LBPs), betaine, phenolics, carotenoids (zeaxanthin and β-carotene), cerebroside, 2-O-β-d-glucopyranosyl-l-ascorbic acid (AA-2βG), β-sitosterol, flavonoids and vitamins, in particular riboflavin, thiamine, and ascorbic acid.[22]

All these compounds are known to support a healthy body and various organ functions. The ingestion of Ningxia wolfberries has also been attributed towards longevity, and this plant is considered one of the superfruits in antiaging medicine.

In fact, the number of centennials in the population living in the valley where most of the Ningxia wolfberries are grown and consumed is significantly higher than in the rest of China. Specifically, 80 persons per million people in that area are over 100 years old compared to only 5 persons per million in the rest of China.[23]

Other health benefits of the Ningxia wolfberry reported in the medical literature include abdominal fat and waist circumference reduction as well as improvement of metabolic profiles,[24] improved function of the eyes,[25,26] improved blood sugar levels in diabetics,[27] improved function of the immune system,[28,29] improved cardiovascular function,[30] improved brain and cognitive function,[31] and even anticancer activities.[32]

In the 1990s, D. Gary Young travelled to the Ningxia region in China and met with an old Chinese doctor. They discussed the fact that so many in that region lived healthily to an old age. The Chinese doctor attributed this partly to the high consumption of Ningxia wolfberries.

Gary was fascinated with this information and started to research this superfruit. He summarized his findings in the book *Ningxia Wolfberry: The Ultimate Superfood* and then began creating different versions of what he originally called Young Berry Juice, which ultimately became today's NingXia Red® drink.

Newer technologies have also allowed the research community to better analyze the ingredients of the Ningxia wolfberry and how they interact on a molecular level. All of this confirms Gary's innate "knowing" about the previously unknown health benefits of the Ningxia wolfberries. And not only is NingXia Red® a great wellness-supporting dietary supplement, it also has a fantastic taste.

As a physician, I know that most people have nutritional deficiencies, depending on various factors such as diet, geographical location, and overall lifestyle. The need for good nutritional elements and antioxidants is like transportation: If you are going through life at a moderate speed, it is like riding a bicycle.

Your bike needs two wheels— you need two NingXia Red® bottles a month. However, if you have an increased need for these compounds due to either a completely sedentary lifestyle or incomplete nutrition, or due to high physical activity in your life, you need four wheels like a car— four bottles of NingXia Red® per month.

Either way, the fact that NingXia Red® is still one of Young Living's bestselling products after almost three decades underlines the popularity and the importance of this drink.

Because of this overwhelming research and information, I recommend adding at least two bottles of NingXia Red® to each month of your Essential Rewards orders. Try NingXia Red® for 30 days and find out for yourself why so many people of all ages consume this product month after month.

Note: None of the statements made about any of Young Living's products have been evaluated by the Food and Drug Administration. Young Living products are not intended to diagnose, treat, cure, or prevent any disease.

Most of the product information and text describing Young Living products is directly from Young Living Essential Oils, LC, and can be found online at youngliving.com

NingXia Red® is a registered trademark of Young Living Essential Oils, LC.

References:

[17] Free Radicals, Antioxidants in Disease and Health. Int J Biomed Sci. 2008 Jun; 4(2): 89–96. PMID: 23675073.

[18] Free radicals and antioxidants in normal physiological functions and human disease. Int J Biochem Cell Biol. 2007;39(1):44-84. PMID: 16978905 DOI: 10.1016/j.biocel.2006.07.001.

[19] Antioxidants to slow aging, facts and perspectives. Presse Med. 2002 Jul 27;31(25):1174-84. PMID: 12192730.

[20] Lycium Barbarum: A Traditional Chinese Herb and A Promising Anti-Aging Agent. Aging Dis. 2017 Dec; 8(6): 778–791. 10.14336/AD.2017.0725.

[21] Lycium barbarum (goji) juice improves in vivo antioxidant biomarkers in serum of healthy adults. Nutr Res. 2009 Jan;29(1):19-25. doi: 10.1016/j.nutres.2008.11.005.

[22] Use of anti-aging herbal medicine, Lycium barbarum, against aging-associated diseases. What do we know so far? Cell Mol Neurobiol. 2008 Aug;28(5):643-52. PMID: 17710531 DOI: 10.1007/s10571-007-9181-x.

[23] Ethnic Living Habit Conductive for Longevity. http://www.china.org.cn/english/culture/110129.htm

[24] Lycium barbarum Reduces Abdominal Fat and Improves Lipid Profile and Antioxidant Status in Patients with Metabolic Syndrome. Oxid Med Cell Longev. 2017; 2017: 9763210. doi: 10.1155/2017/9763210.

[25] Effects of Lycium barbarum on the Visual System. Int Rev Neurobiol. 2017;135:1-27. doi: 10.1016/bs.irn.2017.02.002.

[26] Effects of Lycium barbarum (goji berry) on dry eye disease in rats. Mol Med Rep. 2018 Jan; 17(1): 809–818. doi: 10.3892/mmr.2017.7947.

[27] Practical Application of Antidiabetic Efficacy of Lycium barbarum Polysaccharide in Patients with Type 2 Diabetes. Med Chem. 2015 Jun; 11(4): 383–390. doi: 10.2174/1573406410666141110153858.

[28] Biomolecular and Clinical Aspects of Chinese Wolfberry. Herbal Medicine: Biomolecular and Clinical Aspects, Chapter 14. CRC Press/Taylor & Francis; 2011.

[29] Immunomodulatory effects of a standardized Lycium barbarum fruit juice in Chinese older healthy human subjects. J Med Food. 2009 Oct;12(5):1159-65. doi: 10.1089/jmf.2008.0300.

[30] Protective effect of Lycium barbarum on doxorubicin-induced cardiotoxicity. Phytother Res. 2007 Nov;21(11):1020-4. PMID: 17622973

DOI: 10.1002/ptr.2186.

[31] A milk-based wolfberry preparation prevents prenatal stress-induced cognitive impairment of offspring rats, and inhibits oxidative damage and mitochondrial dysfunction in vitro. Neurochem Res. 2010 May;35(5):702-11. doi: 10.1007/s11064-010-0123-5.

[32] A review of the anticancer and immunomodulatory effects of Lycium barbarum fruit. Inflammopharmacology. 2012 Dec;20(6):307-14. doi: 10.1007/s10787-011-0107-3.

Making the Change

❧CHAPTER 4

Month 1: A Fresh Start

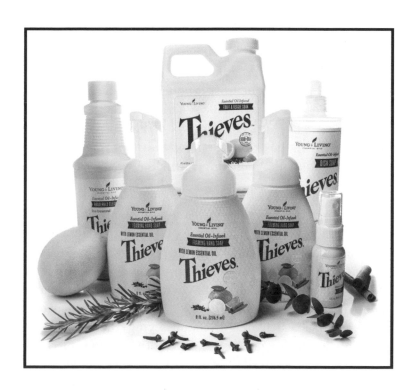

Very few people in the world today understand the incredibly toxic and destructive consequences hiding inside ordinary household cleaning products seen on store shelves everywhere. A 2015 survey estimated that individuals discharge almost 33 liters of chemical products per year down the drain. Dishwashing liquids and hand soaps accounted for 40% of this volume.[33] Once these chemicals wash down the drain and find their way into bodies of water, they impact the environment and wildlife.[34]

But these harsh chemicals also negatively impact the human body.[35,36,37] Another study investigated volatile organic compounds (VOCs) emitted from 25 common fragranced consumer products such as cleaning supplies, personal care products, laundry products, and air fresheners.[38] The study found that each of these products, even so-called "green" or "eco-friendly" products, contained dangerous chemicals labeled toxic or hazardous under U.S. federal laws.

Unfortunately, U.S. regulations do not require disclosure of all ingredients in a consumer product, or of any ingredients in a mixture called "fragrance." A single synthetic fragrance in a product can contain hundreds of chemicals, some of which react with the ozone in ambient air to form dangerous secondary pollutants, including formaldehyde.[39]

In fact, one study shows that women cleaning at home or working as occupational cleaners had an accelerated decline in lung function due to the exposure to the toxins in the commercially available cleaning products. The effect of cleaning was thus comparable to smoking slightly less than 20 pack-years which correlates with moderate to heavy smoking.[40] "Pack-years" quantifies the amount someone smokes and is calculated by multiplying the number of packs of cigarettes smoked per day by the number of years the person has smoked. Twenty pack-years could mean smoking one pack per day for 20 years or two packs per day for ten years.

In other words, the daily use of toxic household products to clean your home is as bad as smoking a pack of cigarettes, every day, for 20 years, and it significantly increases your risk for serious lung disease. Frequent use of chemical household cleaners also increases the incidence rate of wheezing and asthma in young children.[41] In addition, these highly toxic products often cause allergic rhinitis (runny nose) and skin rashes.[42,43,44] Forty-two percent of non-professional cleaners use chemical household cleaner sprays weekly to clean their home.

This regular use was associated with higher incidence of asthma symptoms or medication and wheezing. The incidence of physician-diagnosed asthma was significantly higher among those using such sprays at least four days per week.[45] Another study found that lower respiratory tract symptoms of female non-professional domestic cleaners were more common on working days and were predominantly associated with exposure to diluted bleach, degreasing sprays/atomizers, and air fresheners.[46] In contrast, women using environmentally preferable cleaning products had significantly reduced health problems regarding their skin and respiratory systems.[47]

What about those who clean multiple homes every day? Professional cleaners are exposed to over 130 toxic chemicals from commercial chemical household cleaners. These toxins have been identified as an occupational risk for these workers because of increased incidences of reported respiratory effects, such as asthma and asthma-like symptoms.[48] Anyone employed in domestic or commercial cleaning is at increased risk for symptoms of an obstructive lung disease.[49]

Every time I go to the restroom in a hotel or conference center, or in public restrooms, I find antibacterial soaps. The emergence of products containing antibacterial agents into healthy households has escalated from a few dozen in the mid-1990s to more than 700 today.[50]

In September 2017, the Food and Drug Administration (FDA) published the final ruling prohibiting 19 out of 22 chemicals commonly found in antibacterial soaps, also called anti-septic washes, because they were not safe.[51] Banned chemicals included triclosan (mostly in liquid soaps) and triclocarbon (mostly in bar soaps). Unfortunately, the ruling did not include hand sanitizers and wipes.

The director of the FDA's Center for Drug Evaluation and Research (CDER) stated that, "Consumers may think antibacterial washes are more effective at preventing the spread of germs, but we have no scientific evidence that they are any better than plain soap and water," and that "data suggests that antibacterial ingredients may do more harm than good over the long-term."[52]

Other studies confirmed that the use of antibacterial cleaning and hand soap products did not reduce any infectious diseases in these households, or even in public settings.[53,54] In other words, by using these products, you get all the toxic chemicals on and into your body without any benefits in return.

Skin, the largest human organ, is a complex and dynamic ecosystem inhabited by a multitude of micro-organisms.[55] Regular use of antibacterial soap can cause rapid changes in these microbial communities (the "microbiome" of the skin), with the potential for negative effects on your skin health.[56] We now know that antimicrobial drugs and topical applications can alter skin bacterial families in a significant way, and that these alterations can have critical implications for the defense mechanisms of the skin.[57]

This is confirmed by studies demonstrating a higher frequency of allergies, asthma, and eczema in persons who have been raised in an environment that is overly protective against microorganisms, i.e. in a household with regular use of antibacterial, anti-septic, or anti-microbial products.[58]

There is also the concern that the regular use of antibacterial household products and soaps may increase the occurrence of drug-resistant bacterial strains in the environment. However, there does not currently appear to be strong scientific evidence to support this concern.

These massively damaging effects stem not just from what we put on ourselves or use in our household, but also from the chemicals we spray on the food we eat. It is well-known that fruits and vegetables are essential components of a healthy diet. However, research suggests that pesticides in, and on, produce may pose health risks.

Many consumers don't realize that pesticide residues are common on conventionally grown produce. The United States Department of Agriculture (USDA) analyzed and found 230 different pesticides and pesticide breakdown products on thousands of produce samples.[59] In 2018, the Environmental Working Group reported that more than 98% of samples of strawberries, spinach leaves, peaches, nectarines, cherries, and apples tested positive for residue of at least one pesticide. They also showed that a single sample of strawberries may contain up to 20 different pesticides and that spinach samples had, on average, 1.8 times more pesticide residue by weight than any other crop.[60]

Other researchers found that prenatal exposure to such toxic chemicals resulted in lower IQ's of seven-year-old children.[61] We also know that organic foods significantly lower children's dietary exposure to pesticides from fruits and vegetables.[62] It is also possible that a greater intake of high-pesticide residue from fruits and vegetables is associated with a lower probability of clinical pregnancy and live birth. In fact, the probability of clinical pregnancy was decreased by 18% and the probability of live birth was reduced by 26% in women with the highest levels of pesticide exposure.[63]

But the effects of pesticide exposure by fruits and vegetables is not limited to females. For men, it seems that the intake of fruit and vegetables with high pesticide residues is associated with poorer semen quality. Males with a higher exposure had a 49% lower total sperm count and a 32% lower number of normal sperm than men with less exposure.[64]

Many sources recommend to only use water to wash your fruits and vegetables or to soak the produce for a while in other chemicals such as commercial chlorine bleach. In contrast, Young Living has formulated household cleaners, soaps, and fruit and vegetable washes to be free of harsh chemicals by using a variety of essential oils instead. These natural options are part of the Thieves® line of products.

Young Living's natural cleaning and soap products are based on their Thieves® Essential Oil blend, which contains Lemon, Clove, Eucalyptus, Cinnamon Bark, and Rosemary Essential Oils.

The original blend of four oils goes back to the Middle Ages, during the time of the Black Plague, when it was known as "Marseille Water" or "Marseille Vinegar."[65] Supposedly, robbers used it to protect themselves against the "Black Death" while looting corpses, and hence the name "Thieves." French authorities recognized that there was such value in this mixture that upon the thieves' capture, they offered a more merciful punishment if the thieves divulged the ingredients in their secret formula.

Some tales mention as few as four thieves, while others mention groups of up to 60. The specific blend of essential oils used also varies, but the four most commonly reported essential oils or plant extracts are rosemary, lemon, clove, and cinnamon. Gary Young used these four plants as a starting point and added Eucalyptus Essential Oil to improve the blend. Since then, an entire line of Thieves® products has been created.

It is now very clear why you should get rid of as many toxic chemicals in your household and your personal care products as possible. And thanks to Gary's vision, Young Living has clean alternatives for your household.

Thieves® Household Cleaner

Thieves® Household Cleaner is a concentrated, versatile solution that gives you a deep clean when scrubbing, degreasing, spot cleaning, dusting, and more, all without harsh chemicals. The fact that it is formulated without any severe or dangerous chemicals found in many traditional cleaning products also means that this product has no synthetic chemical smell. It has a fresh and inviting scent. It is safe to use around everyone in your family, including your infants and pets. This plant-based, vegan-friendly, ultra-concentrated, and versatile formula is perfect for virtually every surface in your home including carpets, floors, counters, glass, walls, and more. It uses the typical Thieves® Essential Oil blend containing Clove, Rosemary, Lemon, Cinnamon Bark, and Eucalyptus.

Before using this product, perform a spot test in an inconspicuous area. If staining or damage occurs, discontinue use on the material. Since the Thieves® Household Cleaner is ultraconcentrated, it should be diluted with water before use. And because it can be diluted, one bottle will last much longer than conventional products bought in a store.

Thieves® Foaming Hand Soap

The instant foam produced by Thieves® Foaming Hand Soap makes it easy to lather and rinse your hands. This product combines the Thieves® Essential Oil blend with additional Lemon and Orange Essential Oils, as well as other naturally derived ingredients such as Gingko, Tea Extract, and Aloe to clean your hands. It contains no sulfates, dyes, synthetic fragrances, or harsh chemicals.

Thieves® Spray

Thieves® Spray is a portable essential oil spray ideal for cleaning small surfaces. Just one small spritz freshens counters, sinks, door handles, toilets, and more using only naturally derived, plant-based ingredients, and the powerful spicy-citrus scent of Thieves® Essential Oil blend. Safe to use around children and pets, and the perfect size to throw in a purse, backpack, or luggage, a bottle of Thieves® Spray is ideal to keep with you wherever you go. The spray uses the typical Thieves® Essential Oil blend containing Clove, Rosemary, Lemon, Cinnamon bark, and Eucalyptus.

Thieves® Fruit & Veggie Soak

Young Living's Fruit & Veggie Soak safely and effectively washes produce with the cleansing power of three exclusive essential oil blends: DiGize, Thieves®, and Purification. Perfect for meal preparation or cleaning larger amounts of produce, add a small amount of Thieves® Fruit & Veggie Soak to a basin of water, then soak, rinse, and enjoy clean fruits and vegetables. This Fruit & Veggie Soak was formulated with the following essential oils: Tarragon, Ginger, Peppermint, Juniper, Fennel, Lemongrass, Clove, Rosemary, Citronella, Anise, Lemon, Patchouli, Cinnamon Bark, Tea Tree, Lavandin, Eucalyptus radiata, Tunisian Myrtle, and Moroccan Myrtle.

Thieves® Waterless Hand Purifier

The Thieves® Waterless Hand Purifier is a convenient, portable, and long-lasting waterless hand sanitizer formulated without any toxins. It uses the typical Thieves® Essential Oil blend containing Clove, Rosemary, Lemon, Cinnamon Bark, and Eucalyptus Essential Oils, and is also enhanced with natural Peppermint Essential Oil to better cleanse and purify hands.

Thieves® Dish Soap

Thieves® Dish Soap was formulated with naturally derived ingredients to effectively clean your dishes without chemicals, dyes, or synthetics. In addition to the Thieves® Essential Oil blend containing Clove, Rosemary, Lemon, Cinnamon Bark, and Eucalyptus, this dish soap also includes Jade Lemon and Bergamot Essential Oils. This plant-based formula is free from SLS (sodium lauryl sulfate), SLES (sodium lauryl ether sulfate), dyes, formaldehyde, phosphates, and synthetic perfumes.

It is time to minimize this negative footprint on your body and on our environment. Replace your household products containing toxins and harsh chemicals with essential oil-based options that are friendly to you and the environment.

Note: None of the statements made about any of Young Living's products have been evaluated by the Food and Drug Administration. Young Living products are not intended to diagnose, treat, cure, or prevent any disease.

Most of the product information and text describing Young Living products is directly from Young Living Essential Oils, LC, and can be found online at youngliving. com

KidScents® and Thieves® are registered trademarks of Young Living Essential Oils, LC.

Month 1 Shopping List:

Product Name	Item Number	PV
Thieves® Foaming Hand Soap - 3 pk	3643	36.5
Thieves® Household Cleaner	3743	22.5
Thieves® Spray	3265	9.25
Thieves® Fruit & Veggie Soak	5352	19.75
Thieves® Waterless Hand Purifier	3621	5
Thieves® Dish Soap	5350	14
	Total PV:	107
Bonus Essential Oil: Tea Tree (Melaleuca Alternifolia)		
For Your Kiddo: KidScents® Bath Gel		
Month 1 ER Points Earning Rate: 10%		
Rewards Points Earned this Month:		~10
Cumulative Reward Points:		~10

References:

[33] An Approach for Prioritizing "Down-the-Drain" Chemicals Used in the Household. Int J Environ Res Public Health. 2015 Feb; 12(2): 1351–1367. doi: 10.3390/ijerph120201351.

[34] A review of personal care products in the aquatic environment: environmental concentrations and toxicity. Chemosphere. 2011 Mar;82(11):1518-32. doi: 10.1016/j.chemosphere.2010.11.018.

[35] Toxic effects of the easily avoidable phthalates and parabens. Altern Med Rev. 2010 Sep;15(3):190-6. PMID: 21155623.

[36] Cosmetics as source of xenoestrogens exposure. Przegl Lek. 2013;70(8):647-51.

[37] Environmental oestrogens, cosmetics and breast cancer. Best Pract Res Clin Endocrinol Metab. 2006 Mar;20(1):121-43. PMID: 16522524 DOI: 10.1016/j.beem.2005.09.007.

[38] Fragranced consumer products: Chemicals emitted, ingredients unlisted. Environmental Impact Assessment Review. Volume 31, Issue 3, April 2011, Pages 328-333. doi.org/10.1016/j.eiar.2010.08.002.

[39] Indoor Air Quality: Scented Products Emit a Bouquet of VOCs. Environ Health Perspect. 2011 Jan; 119(1): A16. doi: 10.1289/ehp.119-a16.

[40] Cleaning at home and at work in relation to lung function decline and airway obstruction. Am J Respir Crit Care Med. 2018 May 1;197(9):1157-1163. doi: 10.1164/rccm.201706-1311OC.

[41] Frequent use of chemical household products is associated with persistent wheezing in pre-school age children. Thorax. 2005 Jan; 60(1): 45–49. doi: 10.1136/thx.2004.021154.

[42] Frequent use of household cleaning products is associated with rhinitis in Chinese children. J Allergy Clin Immunol. 2016 Sep;138(3):754-760.e6. doi: 10.1016/j.jaci.2016.03.038.

[43] Association between exposure to antimicrobial household products and allergic symptoms. Environ Health Toxicol. 2014; 29: e2014017. doi: 10.5620/eht.e2014017.

[44] Hazardous substances in frequently used professional cleaning products. Int J Occup Environ Health. 2014 Mar; 20(1): 46–60. doi: 10.1179/2049396713Y.0000000052.

[45] The Use of Household Cleaning Sprays and Adult Asthma. Am J Respir Crit Care Med. 2007 Oct 15; 176(8): 735–741. doi: 10.1164/rccm.200612-1793OC.

[46] Short-term respiratory effects of cleaning exposures in female domestic cleaners. Eur Respir J. 2006 Jun;27(6):1196-203. DOI: 10.1183/09031936.06.00085405.

[47] Traditional and environmentally preferable cleaning product exposure and health symptoms in custodians. Am J Ind Med. 2015 Sep; 58(9): 988–995. doi: 10.1002/ajim.22484.

[48] Characterization of occupational exposures to cleaning products used for common cleaning tasks--a pilot study of hospital cleaners. Environ Health. 2009 Mar 27;8:11. doi: 10.1186/1476-069X-8-11.

[49] Asthma, chronic bronchitis, and exposure to irritant agents in occupational domestic cleaning: a nested case-control study. Occup Environ Med. 2005 Sep;62(9):598-606. DOI: 10.1136/oem.2004.017640.

[50] Antibacterial household products: cause for concern. Emerg Infect Dis. 2001; 7(3 Suppl): 512–515. PMID: 11485643.

[51] The US Food and Drug Administration FDA. Safety and Effectiveness of Consumer Antiseptics; Topical Antimicrobial Drug Products for Over-the-Counter Human Use. https://www.federalregister.gov/documents/2016/09/06/2016-21337/safety-and-effectiveness-of-consumer-antiseptics-topical-antimicrobial-drug-products-for.

[52] FDA issues final rule on safety and effectiveness of antibacterial soaps. Rule removes triclosan and triclocarban from over-the-counter antibacterial hand and body washes. https://www.fda.gov/newsevents/newsroom/pressannouncements/ucm517478.htm.

[53] Effect of Antibacterial Home Cleaning and Handwashing Products on Infectious Disease Symptoms. Ann Intern Med. 2004 Mar 2; 140(5): 321–329.

PMID: 14996673.

[54] Consumer Antibacterial Soaps: Effective or Just Risky? Clinical Infectious Diseases, Volume 45, Issue Supplement_2, 1 September 2007, Pages S137–S147, https://doi.org/10.1086/519255.

[55] Skin microbiota: Microbial community structure and its potential association with health and disease. Infect Genet Evol. 2011 Jul; 11(5): 839–848. doi: 10.1016/j.meegid.2011.03.022.

[56] Antibacterial soap use impacts skin microbial communities in rural Madagascar. PLoS One. 2018; 13(8): e0199899. doi: 10.1371/journal.pone.0199899.

[57] Topical Antimicrobial Treatments Can Elicit Shifts to Resident Skin Bacterial Communities and Reduce Colonization by Staphylococcus aureus Competitors. Antimicrob Agents Chemother. 2017 Sep; 61(9): e00774-17. doi: 10.1128/AAC.00774-17.

[58] Give us this day our daily germs. Immunol Today. 1998 Mar;19(3):113-6. PMID: 9540269.

[59] U.S. Department of Agriculture, Economic Issues in the Coexistence of Organic, Genetically Engineered (GE), and Non-GE Crops. Economic Research Service, 2016. www.ers.usda.gov/webdocs/publications/eib149/56750_eib-149.pdf.

[60] Environmental Working Group EWG. EWG's 2018 Shopper's Guide to Pesticides in Produce. https://www.ewg.org/foodnews/summary.php.

[61] Prenatal exposure to organophosphate pesticides and IQ in 7-year-old children. Environ Health Perspect. 2011 Aug;119(8):1189-95. doi: 10.1289/ehp.1003185.

[62] Organic Diets Significantly Lower Children's Dietary Exposure to Organophosphorus Pesticides. Environ Health Perspect. 2006 Feb; 114(2): 260–263. doi: 10.1289/ehp.8418.

[63] Association Between Pesticide Residue Intake From Consumption of Fruits and Vegetables and Pregnancy Outcomes Among Women Undergoing Infertility Treatment With Assisted Reproductive Technology. JAMA Intern Med. 2018 Jan 1;178(1):17-26. doi: 10.1001/jamainternmed.2017.5038.

[64] Fruit and vegetable intake and their pesticide residues in relation to semen quality among men from a fertility clinic. Hum Reprod. 2015 Jun;30(6):1342-51. doi: 10.1093/humrep/dev064.

[65] Paris, Pharmacologia, 1825. https://books.google.com/books?id=B5k-AAAAYAAJ&lpg=PA242&ots= MDTOOTup-D&dq=paris,%20pharmacologia,%206th%20edit&pg=PA18#v=onepage&q=four%20thieves&f=false.

⚘CHAPTER 5

Month 2: Teeth & Sheets

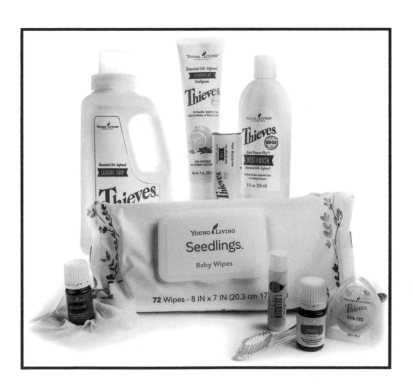

Have you ever thought about the chemicals you absorb through your mouth every day? Regular commercial toothpastes contain a variety of chemicals, fluoride being the most well-known. We are exposed to fluoride from drinking water, fluoridated dental products, and cleaning products. Water fluoridation represents 30% to 70% of a typical individual's total exposure. Fluoride is added to municipal water supplies and dental products, such as toothpaste, to prevent or reduce tooth decay.[66] It is well-established that by brushing our teeth at least once a day with a fluoride-containing toothpaste, there will be less tooth decay.[67]

The use of fluoride, especially in children with developing brains, has recently been questioned. Fluoride is a well-known neurotoxin.[68] Several studies showed that children exposed to fluoride had a lower IQ and suffered impairment in neurological development.[69,70]

When the impact of human exposure to fluoride from municipal water and dental products was tested, it was shown that the microbiome of the oral cavity (mouth), but not the microbiome of the gut, underwent significant changes by depleting some important microbiotic strains.[71] It is not yet known whether these fluoride-related changes will impact oral, neurological, or cardiovascular health.

Though the scientific discussion is still ongoing and no good study currently exists on the effects of toothpaste-related fluoride exposure as correlated to neurological impairment, based on what we do know, common sense tells us that fluoride should be avoided especially when natural alternatives for dental hygiene already exist.

Furthermore, several toothpastes contain chlorhexidine or triclosan, chemicals used in many consumer products to reduce or prevent bacterial contamination. It was found that triclosan accumulates on your toothbrush and is then released into your mouth in an uncontrollable manner.[72] In a ruling effective mid-2017, the FDA finally banned triclosan from all over-the-counter products unless sufficient evidence is provided regarding their efficacy and safety.[73] If used, triclosan now has to be disclosed on the label as an active ingredient.

Other potentially harmful ingredients of toothpastes include sodium lauryl sulfate (SLS), artificial sweeteners, propylene glycol, diethanolamine (DEA), artificial coloring agents, and microbeads. Microbeads are tiny plastic spheres that were introduced in the 1970s into many of our daily products.

Today, they represent a significant part of the plastic accumulation on Planet Earth since they are flushed down our drains and then pollute the waters. Microbeads have been reported in every major ocean and many lakes and waterways. By ending up in these aquatic habitats, they made it into our food chain and we now consume and absorb these microplastics not only via cleaning and personal care products, but also via food.[74] Luckily, many states in the US as well as other countries around the world are finally in the process of banning the use of microbeads.

Toothpaste containing natural ingredients such as Australian Melaleuca Alternifolia essential oil and ethanolic extract of Polish propolis (from honeybees) improved oral hygiene and the microbiome in the mouth.[75] Function-structure claims regarding known supplements or food, like honey, citing the appropriate references in scientific literature are permitted (at least in the U.S.).

Another study demonstrated the beneficial effect that peppermint or eucalyptus essential oils can have on oral hygiene.[76] Furthermore, the oral use of clove extract can reduce the growth of oral pathogens.[77] The same effect can be demonstrated when using peppermint, tea tree, or thyme essential oils.[78] In addition, the oral use of tea tree essential oils demonstrated a reduction in oral plaque formation.[79]

Keep in mind that your mouth has an incredibly high and fast absorption rate. So why would you want to use this chemical brew called "regular" toothpaste? Make a smarter choice for your body and the environment by switching immediately to Young Living dental products, which are formulated without toxins. And add them to future Essential Rewards orders as you start running out, so that you never have to live without these better options.

Thieves® AromaBright™ Toothpaste

Thieves® AromaBright™ Toothpaste has naturally derived ingredients formulated to support healthy-looking gums and teeth, remove stains, gently brush away daily buildup, and provide long-lasting fresh breath. It provides a refreshing minty taste with 100% pure essential oils. Added to this toothpaste is the Thieves® Essential Oil blend with essential oils of Clove, Lemon, Cinnamon Bark, Eucalyptus, and Rosemary.

In addition, Peppermint, Ocotea, and Spearmint Essential Oils were added for freshness. This product is formulated without toxins and does not have sulfates, synthetic dyes, artificial flavors, nor preservatives. With AromaBright™ you can ditch the ingredients in commercial toothpastes you don't want and keep all the results you do want: deeply cleaned and bright teeth and fresh breath.

Thieves® Fresh Essence Mouthwash™

Thieves® Fresh Essence Mouthwash™ provides fresh breath and supports healthy-looking gums and teeth. It combines the spicy-sweet flavor of the Thieves® Essential Oil blend (including Clove, Lemon, Cinnamon Bark, Eucalyptus, and Rosemary Essential Oils), Spearmint, Vetiver, and Peppermint Essential Oils, and soap bark tree extract as well as Stevia leaves to give you fresh breath and a pleasant taste in your mouth. This mouthwash is free from harsh alcohol, artificial dyes, and synthetic flavors.

Thieves® Dental Floss™

Thieves® Dental Floss™ was made with strong fibers that resist fraying and easily glide between teeth. Saturated twice, this hard-wearing floss provides two layers of essential oils, offering double the protection to freshen your breath. The essential oils used to saturate the fibers are Clove, Lemon, Cinnamon Bark, Eucalyptus, and Rosemary.

Lavender Lip Balm

I also suggest adding Lavender Lip Balm to your Month 2 order. When talking about teeth, we should also look at the products used around your mouth, namely lip products. Unfortunately, many lip products contain heavy metals such as lead.[80] Lead was detected in 75% of the lip products.[81]Most of the tested lip products contained high concentrations of titanium and aluminum. All of them had detectable manganese. Lavender Lip Balm takes advantage of the power of Lavender Essential Oil and the moisturizing and soothing properties of jojoba oil, beeswax, and vitamin E. Treat your lips well and use naturally derived products.

Orange Vitality™ Essential Oil

A 2010 study looked at the effect of d-limonene on 408 subjects, 201 with smoking stains and 207 with tea stains. The results were impressive. Five percent d-limonene, combined with whitening formulation, significantly reduced stain scores both for smoking stain removal and inhibition. The five percent d-limonene alone exhibited an advantage for smoking stain inhibition.[82] D-limonene is commonly found in lemons, limes, and especially oranges. Because of the acidity of these fruits, it is not advised to use the juice or fruit to make teeth appear whiter.

Orange Vitality™ Essential Oil, however, does not contain the acidity levels of the fruit itself. In addition, the rinds of citrus fruits contain more d-limonene than the pulp or juice, and Orange Vitality™ Essential Oil is made by cold-pressing orange rinds. As you get more comfortable with using essential oils, I recommend putting a drop of Orange Vitality™ Essential Oil on your natural toothpaste every once in a while to make your teeth appear whiter.

Thieves® Mints

Thieves® Mints were created as healthy alternative to freshen your breath without using any synthetic fragrances. This product was formulated by Young Living using Clove, Lemon, Cinnamon Bark, Eucalyptus, and Rosemary Essential Oils. In addition, Peppermint Essential Oil was added to give your mouth a refreshing feeling. Even better news: Thieves® Mints are sugar-free.

But wait - your dental products are only half the battle for this month. The other category we are tackling with your Month 2 order is your laundry room. Here's why:

Typical laundry soaps contain surfactants, builders, bleaching agents, enzymes, brighteners, artificial fragrances, and other ingredients to remove dirt, stain, and soil from surfaces or textiles and to give them a pleasant feel and odor. Optical brighteners are used to make clothes appear more vibrant, which has nothing to do with cleaning clothes. Clothes only appear whiter and brighter because these additives reflect blue light, giving the illusion that your clothes are less yellow. Once washed and dried, clothes and other textiles contaminated with these toxins will come in contact with the skin.

Over the past decade or so, there have been substantial pushes in medicine to better understand the human microbiome and its importance for immune defense and brain development and function, as well as other important physiological functions of the body.

We are on the verge of understanding the negative impacts of chemicals, antibiotics, and toxins on the development and maintenance of a healthy bacterial population on and within our bodies. It is likely that the ambient environment has an important effect on developing the microbiome of the skin (stratabiome), including contact with detergents and hygienic products, soaps, moisturizers, and cosmetics.[83] The degree of detergent use was identified to be one of the factors that can dramatically alter the surface environment of the skin.[84] Thus, the microbiome will also be influenced.

And an altered skin microbiome could have disastrous effect on the immune system.[85] Research demonstrated the profound reliance of the skin's immune system on the skin bacteria for both host defense and tissue repair.[86] Current science recognizes the intricate interactions of microbes and immune cells on the skin surface.[87] In fact, having beneficial bacteria on the skin is so important that recent studies confirmed the positive effect pre- and probiotics can have when applied to the skin.[88]

Equipped with this knowledge, we should ask ourselves what the consequences are when clothes washed with highly toxic chemicals touch us and come in contact with the skin's microbiome. In my mind, such contact should be avoided whenever possible. Why even consider using toxic laundry detergents full with harsh chemicals when better alternatives exist?

Thieves® Laundry Soap

With a plant-based formula, Thieves® Laundry Soap gently and naturally washes your clothes and cleans them without any chemical or synthetic residue. Natural enzymes and powerful essential oils add to the formula's strength to leave your clothes fresh and clean with a light citrus scent. Thieves® Laundry Soap can be used in all washers including high-efficiency washing machines.

Its highly concentrated formula (6X) will provide around 64 loads with just 32 fl. oz (946 ml). The essential oils used in this plant-base product include the typical Thieves® Essential Oil blend with Clove, Lemon, Cinnamon Bark, Eucalyptus, and Rosemary Essential Oils. In addition, Jade Lemon and Bergamot Essential Oils were added. This product is formulated without toxins and contains no SLS, dyes, petrochemicals, formaldehyde, phosphates, synthetic perfume, and optical brighteners.

Seedling™ Baby Wipes

Dryer sheets were invented in the late 1960s and contain a thin layer of lubricant which is electronically conductive. Dryer sheets are used to make laundry feel softer and help prevent static cling. It was found that dryer sheets contain a variety of harsh chemicals such as bucinal, HHCB (galaxolide), phthalates, and methyl ionone, AHTN (acetyl hexamethyl tetralin), isobornyl acetate, parabens, bisphenol A (BPA), triclosan, ethanolamines, alkylphenols, fragrances, glycol ethers, cyclosiloxanes, and phenethyl alcohol. One study detected 55 chemical compounds in all fragranced products, especially perfumes, air fresheners, and dryer sheets.

They also noted that many detected chemicals were not listed on product labels.[89] No wonder. Shockingly, current regulations by the United States Consumer Product Safety

Commission do not require dryer sheet manufacturers to list actual ingredients or chemicals used in fragrances. A 2009 study found that about 11% of the U.S. population reported irritation by scented laundry products which were vented outside.[90] A couple of years later, another study found 29 unique volatile organic compounds (VOCs) in dryer-vent emissions.[91] Of these, the U.S. Environmental Protection Agency (EPA) classifies seven compounds (acetaldehyde, benzene, ethylbenzene, methanol, m/p-xylene, o-xylene, and toluene) as hazardous air pollutants.[92] Together with air fresheners, dryer sheets are regarded as some of the most toxic and hazardous products in a household.

You may wonder why I listed Seedlings™ Baby Wipes this month when talking about healthy teeth and sheets. They're not just for babies! Ditch the chemically-laden dryer sheets and switch to Seedlings Baby Wipes. Throw one wipe into the dryer with your clothes or linens for a gentle, clean scent and to reduce static electricity.

Purification® Essential Oil Blend

Air fresheners have been listed as one of the worst airborne toxic products in a home, and there have even been reports of adults passing out when smelling these artificial toxic scents.[93] One study found that 19% of the surveyed U.S. population reported adverse health effects from air fresheners.[94] Unfortunately, there is no law in the U.S. requiring manufacturers to disclose the chemicals used in these fragrances.[95]

The ingredients of air fresheners can react with the ozone to produce secondary pollutants such as formaldehyde, secondary organic aerosol, oxidative product, and ultrafine particles. These chemical pollutants adversely affect human health by causing damage to the central nervous system, changing hormone levels, or increasing allergies and respiratory diseases. The ultrafine particles may induce severe adverse effects on diverse organs including the pulmonary and cardiovascular systems.

Indoor and in-car use of air fresheners is increasing, but deleterious effects do not manifest for a long time, making it difficult to identify air freshener-associated symptoms.[96] Another lesser-known fact is that air fresheners also release considerable amounts of non-odorous solvents and chemical by-products into the air inside your home.[97]

Other authors have likewise noted the presence of chemicals with known irritants and neurotoxic properties in air fresheners. They even concluded that air fresheners may have actually exacerbated indoor air pollution in addition to releasing toxic chemicals into the atmosphere.[98] The Environmental Working Group (EWG) warns that these products can trigger allergies and often contain suspected endocrine disruptors, such as phthalates and synthetic musks.[99] The EWG also recommends avoiding air fresheners as well as scented cleaning or laundry products that don't disclose their fragrance ingredients on the product label. Please stop using chemically-laden products and turn to natural options, like diffusers and 100% pure, therapeutic-grade essential oils.

Purification®, a blend of six essential oils, is the ultimate weapon against odors. Citronella, Lavandin, Lemongrass, Rosemary, Myrtle, and Tea Tree work together to create a refreshing, bright scent that keeps you and your family happy and comfortable. Purification® clears the air of unwanted odors and freshens musty and stale areas with its lively scent.

Use it around the house, office, and in the car. Diffuse Purification® Essential Oil after cooking, in rooms that smell like your pets, in musty smelling cellars or attics, in air vents, in the garage, in the gym (use a drop or two in the gym bag or add a cotton ball with it into your gym shoes), in kids' rooms that need a little pick-me-up, to freshen your armpits (be sure to dilute), and anywhere else to obtain a pleasant, fresh scent. You can also add a few drops to your Young Living Dryer Balls or Thieves® Laundry Soap to give your laundry a bright-smelling boost.

Many also topically apply this oil blend to soothe the skin after a visit from outdoor annoyances. And because of the known effects of Citronella and Lemongrass, filling an area with the aroma of Purification may keep those bugs a little further away from you and your loved ones.

Don't use any air toxic and dangerous fresheners when you have healthy alternatives at hand. With the scent of Purification® Essential Oil in the air, you'll never need to endanger your family with harsh chemicals from "normal" air fresheners.

Note: None of the statements made about any of Young Living's products have been evaluated by the Food and Drug Administration. Young Living products are not intended to diagnose, treat, cure, or prevent any disease.

Most of the product information and text describing Young Living products is directly from Young Living Essential Oils, LC, and can be found online at youngliving.com

Spearmint Vitality™, KidScents®, Thieves®, AromaBright™, Orange Vitality™, Seedlings™, and Purification® are trademarks of Young Living Essential Oils, LC.

Month 2 Shopping List:

Product Name	Item Number	PV
Thieves® Laundry Soap	5349	29.5
Purification® Essential Oil 5ml	3389	15.75
Baby Wipes - YL Seedlings™ Single	20428	7
Thieves® Dental Floss 1 ct	4463122	3.25
Thieves® Fresh Essence Mouthwash	3683	11.25
Lavender Lip Balm	5203	4
Thieves® AromaBright™ Toothpaste	3039	10.5
Orange Vitality™ - 5ml	5627	6
Thieves® Mints	5138	13
	Total PV:	100.25
Bonus Essential Oil: Spearmint Vitality™ - 5 ml		
For Your Kiddo: KidScents® Slique Toothpaste 114g		
Month 2 ER Points Earning Rate: 10%		
Rewards Points Earned this Month:		~10
Cumulative Reward Points:		~20

References:

[66] Fluoride: Potential Developmental Neurotoxicity. National Toxicology Program. https://ntp.niehs.nih.gov/pubhealth/hat/selected/fluoride/neuro-index.html.

[67] Fluoride toothpastes for preventing dental caries in children and adolescents. Cochrane Database of Systematic Reviews 2003, Issue 1. Art. No.: CD002278. DOI: 10.1002/14651858.CD002278.

[68] Developmental Neurotoxicity of Fluoride: A Quantitative Risk Analysis Toward Establishing a Safe Dose for Children. DOI: 10.5772/intechopen.70852.

[69] Developmental Fluoride Neurotoxicity: A Systematic Review and Meta-Analysis. Environ Health Perspect. 2012 Oct; 120(10): 1362–1368. doi: 10.1289/ehp.1104912.

[70] Effect of fluoride exposure on the intelligence of school children in Madhya Pradesh, India. J Neurosci Rural Pract. 2012 May-Aug; 3(2): 144–149. doi: 10.4103/0976-3147.98213.

[71] Fluoride Depletes Acidogenic Taxa in Oral but Not Gut Microbial Communities in Mice. mSystems. 2017 Jul-Aug; 2(4): e00047-17. doi: 10.1128/mSystems.00047-17.

[72] Nylon Bristles and Elastomers Retain Centigram Levels of Triclosan and Other Chemicals from Toothpastes: Accumulation and Uncontrolled Release. Environ. Sci. Technol., 2017, 51 (21), pp 12264–12273. DOI: 10.1021/acs.est.7b02839.

[73] Safety and Effectiveness of Consumer Antiseptics; Topical Antimicrobial Drug Products for Over-the-Counter Human Use. Docket No. FDA-1975-N-0012 Formerly Part of Docket No. 1975N-0183H.

[74] Scientific Evidence Supports a Ban on Microbeads. https://pubs.acs.org/doi/pdfplus/10.1021/acs.est.5b03909. 2018.

[75] The Influence of Toothpaste Containing Australian Melaleuca alternifolia Oil and Ethanolic Extract of Polish Propolis on Oral Hygiene and Microbiome in Patients Requiring Conservative Procedures. Molecules. 2017 Nov 13;22(11). pii: E1957. doi: 10.3390/molecules22111957.

[76] The effect of Mentha spicata and Eucalyptus camaldulensis essential oils on dental biofilm. Send to Int J Dent Hyg. 2009 Aug;7(3):196-203. doi: 10.1111/j.1601-5037.2009.00389.x.

[77] Compounds from Syzygium aromaticum possessing growth inhibitory activity against oral pathogens. J Nat Prod. 1996 Oct;59(10):987-90. DOI: 10.1021/np960451q.

[78] Antimicrobial efficacy of five essential oils against oral pathogens: An in vitro study. Eur J Dent. 2013 Sep; 7(Suppl 1): S71–S77. doi: 10.4103/1305-7456.119078.

[79] The Antiplaque Efficacy of Two Herbal-Based Toothpastes: A Clinical Intervention. J Int Soc Prev Community Dent. 2018 Jan-Feb; 8(1): 21–27. doi: 10.4103/jispcd.JISPCD_411_17.

[80] Metals in Lip Products - A Cause for Concern? Environ Health Perspect. 2013 Jun; 121(6): a196. doi: 10.1289/ehp.121-a196.

[81] Concentrations and Potential Health Risks of Metals in Lip Products. Environ Health Perspect. 2013 Jun; 121(6): 705–710. doi: 10.1289/ehp.1205518.

[82] Effect of toothpaste containing d-limonene on natural extrinsic smoking stain: a 4-week clinical trial. Am J Dent. 2010 Aug;23(4):196-200. PMID: 21250568.

[83] The skin microbiome: impact of modern environments on skin ecology, barrier integrity, and systemic immune programming. World Allergy Organ J. 2017; 10(1): 29. doi: 10.1186/s40413-017-0160-5.

[84] Functions of the skin microbiota in health and disease. Semin Immunol. 2013 Nov 30; 25(5): 370–377. doi: 10.1016/j.smim.2013.09.005.

[85] Skin Immune Landscape: Inside and Outside the Organism. Mediators

Inflamm. 2017; 2017: 5095293. doi: 10.1155/2017/5095293.

[86] The influence of skin microorganisms on cutaneous immunity. Nat Rev Immunol. 2016 May 27;16(6):353-66. doi: 10.1038/nri.2016.48.

[87] Dialogue between skin microbiota and immunity. Science. 2014 Nov 21;346(6212):954-9. doi: 10.1126/science.1260144.

[88] Impact of prebiotics and probiotics on skin health. Benef Microbes. 2014 Jun 1;5(2):99-107. doi: 10.3920/BM2013.0040.

[89] Endocrine Disruptors and Asthma-Associated Chemicals in Consumer Products. Environ Health Perspect. 2012 Jul; 120(7): 935–943. doi: 10.1289/ehp.1104052.

[90] Prevalence of fragrance sensitivity in the American population. J Environ Health. 2009 Mar;71(7):46-50. PMID: 19326669.

[91] Dryer Vents: An Overlooked Source of Pollution? Environ Health Perspect. 2011 Nov; 119(11): a474–a475. doi: 10.1289/ehp.119-a474a.

[92] U.S. Environmental Protection Agency EPA. Technology Transfer Network. Air Toxics Web Site. Original List of Hazardous Air Pollutant: http://tinyurl.com/yjunv3o.

[93] Indoor Air Quality: Scented Products Emit a Bouquet of VOCs. Environ Health Perspect. 2011 Jan; 119(1): A16. doi: 10.1289/ehp.119-a16.

[94] Prevalence of fragrance sensitivity in the American population. J Environ Health. 2009 Mar;71(7):46-50. PMID: 19326669.

[95] Fragranced consumer products and undisclosed ingredients. Environmental Impact Assess Review. 2009;29(1):32–38. doi: 10.1016/j.eiar.2008.05.002.

[96] Characterization of air freshener emission: the potential health effects. J Toxicol Sci. 2015;40(5):535-50. doi: 10.2131/jts.40.535.

[97] Impact of room fragrance products on indoor air quality. Atmospheric Environment. Volume 106, April 2015, Pages 492-502. doi.org/10.1016/j.atmosenv.2014.11.020.

[98] Toxic effects of air freshener emissions. Arch Environ Health. 1997 Nov-Dec;52(6):433-41. DOI: 10.1080/00039899709602222.

[99] Environmental Working Group EWG. EWG's Healthy Living: Home Guide. https://www.ewg.org/healthyhomeguide/cleaners-and-air-fresheners/#.W7uQ6mhKiUk.

↳CHAPTER 6

Month 3: Lather With Lavender

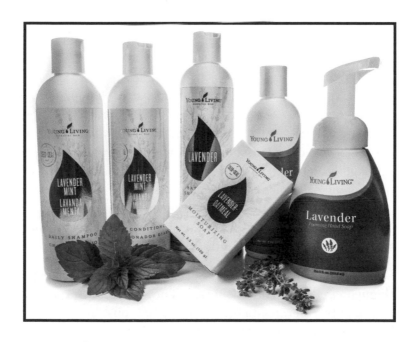

Why watch a scary movie when you can just go read the terrifying labels on everything in your bathroom? Common shower gels, shampoos, and conditioners contain a large amount of potentially damaging ingredients such as detergents, conditioners, thickeners, sequestering agents, pH adjusters, preservatives, and specialty additives. When reading labels, you will often find parabens, synthetic colors, synthetic fragrances, triclosan, sodium lauryl sulfate (SLS), sodium laureth sulfate (SLES), formaldehyde, toluene, and other harsh chemicals.

SLS is a detergent and surfactant found in many personal care products. It is an inexpensive and very effective foaming agent. SLS has been linked to cancer, neurotoxicity, organ toxicity, skin irritation, and endocrine disruption. According to the Environmental Working Group's Skin Deep Cosmetic Safety Database, SLS is a "moderate hazard."[100] It is toxic to aquatic organisms, and it's strongly advised that this substance does not enter the environment.[101] SLES is a related chemical, which has a higher foaming ability and is slightly less irritating than SLS.

So why would you use shower gels and shampoos full of this stuff with the potential to harm yourself and the environment when other, gentler options are available? Also, most people shower with hot water, which opens pores in the skin and scalp. This is the worst time to expose yourself to these dangerous chemicals from harsh commercial products because your absorption of these chemicals is significantly increased. Instead, relax in a hot shower or bath by using soaps and shampoos with natural ingredients.

Young Living offers a variety of gentle shower gels, shampoos, and conditioners. They contain natural ingredients, therapeutic-grade essential oils, no mineral oils, no synthetic perfumes, and no artificial colorings.

Lavender has been used for its benefits for many centuries. The Ancient Greek physician, pharmacologist, and botanist Pedanius Dioscorides praised the many qualities and uses of lavender. Lavender has a calming, soothing, and balancing effect on the mind and skin. Young Living's Lavender Essential Oil is made from lavender (Lavandula angustifolia, also called "English lavender" and "real" or "pure" lavender) grown on two of Young Living's farms, located in Utah and Idaho, and on its partner farm co-op in France. Lavender Essential Oil is steam-distilled from the flowering tops of the plant, and it takes 27 square feet of lavender plants to make one 15-ml bottle of Lavender Essential Oil.[102]

According to Young Living, Lavender Essential Oil promotes feelings of calm, fights occasional nervous tension, has balancing properties that calm the mind and body, cleanses and soothes minor skin irritations, can be soothing to the skin after a day in the sun, reduces the appearance of blemishes, supports aging skin, and includes the naturally occurring constituents linalyl acetate, linalool, and ocimene. Because of these wonderful properties, Young Living created an entire line of natural lavender-infused products.

In the scientific and medical world, lavender (and specifically lavender essential oil) is considered one of the best-selling, over-the-counter herbal remedies for anxiety, stress, and depression. International organizations, such as the World Health Organization (WHO), the European Scientific Cooperative on Phytotherapy (ESCOP), and the European Medicines Agency (EMA) all approve this medicinal plant to relieve stress, restlessness, and anxiety.[103]

Since lavender essential oil has been registered as dietary supplement by Young Living, function-structure claims citing the appropriate references in scientific literature are permitted (at least in the U.S.). Such studies have shown that lavender essential oil displays anti-inflammatory, antioxidant, and analgesic (pain relieving) activity.[104,105] Because of these properties, lavender essential oil has also shown to have neuroprotective effects.[106] It has been used in a variety of clinical settings and even demonstrated a reduction of aggressive behaviors in patients with dementia.[107]

Lavender was also able to improve mild insomnia.[108] In osteoarthritic patients with knee pain, aromatherapy massages with lavender oil resulted in an immediate significant improvement during daily living activities, which continued after the intervention.[109] Essential oils rich in linalool and linalyl acetate, like lavender, also demonstrated a significant beneficial effect on Tension-Anxiety and Anger-Hostility scores in pregnant women.[110]

In surgery settings, lavender aromatherapy reduced preoperative anxiety.[111,112] Lavender aromatherapy also had beneficial effects on intravenous cannulation pain, anxiety, and satisfaction level of patients undergoing surgery.[113] In addition, aromatherapy with lavender essential oil decreases the number of required analgesics following tonsillectomy in pediatric patients.[114] In another clinical postoperative study, patients treated with lavender required half as many opioids and required them about half as often, and it was therefore concluded that lavender aromatherapy can be used to reduce the demand for opioids in the immediate postoperative period.[115]

Similar studies could not show a reduction of pain medication requirement in postoperative care unit settings. However, patients in the lavender aromatherapy group reported a higher satisfaction rate with pain control than patients in the control group.[116] Other studies mentioned that lavender oil has the potential to promote wound healing in the early phase by accelerating the formation of granulation tissue and influencing tissue remodeling via collagen replacement.[117] Lavender essential oil has also shown to promote hair growth.[118] In summary, lavender is a fascinating plant with many beneficial applications. Lavender's calming scent and soothing effects makes it an ideal plant for use in natural personal care products.

Lavender Mint Daily Shampoo and Lavender Mint Daily Conditioner

Lavender Mint Daily Shampoo and Lavender Mint Daily Conditioner are individual products that are formulated to work synergistically together. The shampoo and conditioner provide invigorating daily cleansing and moisturizing suitable for all hair types. Both have key ingredients of Peppermint and Lavender Essential Oils, spearmint leaf extract, panthenol (vitamin B5), hydrolyzed silk, rosemary leaf extract, horsetail extract, Mojave yucca root extract, seaweed extract, Ningxia wolfberry fruit extract, coco-glucoside, rice extract, and algae extract.

Lavender Foaming Hand Soap

Lavender Foaming Hand Soap cleanses and conditions your hands without leaving dryness or irritation. Infused with Lavender Essential Oil, vitamin E, and aloe, this soap is effective and gentle enough for the most sensitive skin. This gentle and great smelling soap has Lavender, Myrrh, and Lemon Essential Oils. Ingredients also include green tea leaf extract, Vitamin A and E, aloe vera, anis, and ginkgo biloba leaf extract. Note: This product also contains corn, soy, and coconut/palm ingredients.

Lavender Bath & Shower Gel

Infused with pure Lavender Essential Oil, Lavender Bath & Shower Gel cleanses, soothes, and relaxes your skin. It's free of chemicals and synthetic preservatives and contains plant-based ingredients such as coconut oil and star anise. This bath & shower gel includes Lavender, Myrrh, Davana, and Lemon Essential Oils. Ingredients also include anis, sea salt, and rosemary extract. Note: This product also contains corn, soy, and coconut/palm ingredients.

Lavender Hand & Body Lotion

Infused with Lavender Essential Oil and other plant-based ingredients, Lavender Hand & Body Lotion moisturizes and protects skin from overexposure for long-lasting hydration. This gentle lotion includes Lavender, Myrrh, Davana, and Lemon Essential Oils. Ingredients also include barley extract, amur cork tree extract, sandalwood extract, oarweed extract, hydrolyzed silk, vitamin E, murumuru butter, wolfberry seed oil, olive fruit oil, and rosemary extract.

Lavender Oatmeal Bar Soap

With a relaxing floral scent and luxuriously creamy formula, Young Living's Lavender Oatmeal Bar Soap leaves skin feeling soft, smooth, and refreshed. Oats offer gentle exfoliation and remove excess oil while moisturizing botanicals such as coconut, jojoba, and wolfberry seed oils and five therapeutic-grade essential oils prevent over-drying. With its 100% vegetable-based formula, this bar is vegan-friendly. It's also hypoallergenic and made without synthetic dyes or colorants, parabens, petrochemicals, or sulfates, so it's gentle enough for all skin types. This great smelling bar soap was created with Lavender, Coriander, Bergamot (furanocoumarin-free), Ylang Ylang, and Geranium Essential Oils. Ingredients also include wolfberry seed oil, oat kernel flour, olive fruit oil, oat bran, jojoba seed oil, oat kernel meal, aloe vera, and rosemary leaf extract. Note: This product also contains corn, soy, and coconut/ palm ingredients.

Month 3 Shopping List:

Product Name	Item Number	PV
Lavender Mint Daily Shampoo	5191121	20.25
Lavender Mint Daily Conditioner	5192121	20.25
Lavender Foaming Hand Soap Single	4430	11.75
Lavender Bath & Shower Gel	5202	19
Lavender Hand & Body Lotion	5201	21.25
Lavender Oatmeal Soap	4904	10.5
	Total PV:	103
Bonus Essential Oil: Valor™		
For Your Kiddo: KidScents® Shampoo		
Month 3 ER Points Earning Rate: 10%		
Rewards Points Earned this Month:		~10
Cumulative Reward Points:		~31

Note: *None of the statements made about any of Young Living's products have been evaluated by the Food and Drug Administration. Young Living products are not intended to diagnose, treat, cure, or prevent any disease.*

Most of the product information and text describing Young Living products is directly from Young Living Essential Oils, LC, and can be found online at youngliving.com

Valor® and KidScents® are registered trademarks of Young Living Essential Oils, LC.

References:

[100] Environmental Working Group's Skin Deep Cosmetic Safety Database. https://www.ewg.org/skindeep/ingredient/706110/SODIUM_LAURYL_SULFATE/#.W3sUCuhKiUk.

[101] The National Institute for Occupational Safety and Health (NIOSH). Center for Disease Control and Prevention CDC. https://www.cdc.gov/niosh/ipcsneng/neng0502.html.

[102] Young Living Lavender Essential Oil Product Information Page. https://static.youngliving.com/en-US/PDFS/PIP-Lavender.pdf.

[103] Exploring Pharmacological Mechanisms of Lavender (Lavandula angustifolia) Essential Oil on Central Nervous System Targets. Front Pharmacol. 2017; 8: 280. doi: 10.3389/fphar.2017.00280.

[104] Effect of Lavender (Lavandula angustifolia) Essential Oil on Acute Inflammatory Response. Evid Based Complement Alternat Med. 2018; 2018: 1413940. doi: 10.1155/2018/1413940.

[105] Antioxidant, analgesic and anti-inflammatory effects of lavender essential oil. An Acad Bras Cienc. 2015 Aug;87(2 Suppl):1397-408. doi: 10.1590/0001-3765201520150056.

[106] Neuroprotective activity of lavender oil on transient focal cerebral ischemia in mice. Molecules. 2012 Aug 15;17(8):9803-17. doi: 10.3390/molecules17089803.

[107] The study protocol of a blinded randomised-controlled cross-over trial of lavender oil as a treatment of behavioural symptoms in dementia. BMC Geriatr. 2010; 10: 49. doi: 10.1186/1471-2318-10-49.

[108] A single-blinded, randomized pilot study evaluating the aroma of Lavandula augustifolia as a treatment for mild insomnia. J Altern Complement Med. 2005 Aug;11(4):631-7. DOI: 10.1089/acm.2005.11.631.

[109] Aromatherapy massage with lavender essential oil and the prevention of disability in ADL in patients with osteoarthritis of the knee: A randomized controlled clinical trial. Complement Ther Clin Pract. 2018 Feb;30:116-121. doi: 10.1016/j.ctcp.2017.12.012.

[110] Physical and Psychologic Effects of Aromatherapy Inhalation on Pregnant Women: A Randomized Controlled Trial. J Altern Complement Med. 2013 Oct; 19(10): 805–810. doi: 10.1089/acm.2012.0103

[111] The Efficacy of Lavender Aromatherapy in Reducing Preoperative Anxiety in Ambulatory Surgery Patients Undergoing Procedures in General Otolaryngology. Laryngoscope Investig Otolaryngol. 2017 Dec; 2(6): 437–441. doi: 10.1002/lio2.121

[112] Both lavender fleur oil and unscented oil aromatherapy reduce preoperative anxiety in breast surgery patients: a randomized trial. J Clin Anesth. 2016 Sep;33:243-9. doi: 10.1016/j.jclinane.2016.02.032.

[113] Evaluating the efficacy of lavender aromatherapy on peripheral venous cannulation pain and anxiety: A prospective, randomized study. Complement Ther Clin Pract. 2016 May;23:64-8. doi: 10.1016/j.ctcp.2016.03.008.

[114] Evaluation of the effect of aromatherapy with lavender essential oil on post-tonsillectomy pain in pediatric patients: a randomized controlled trial. Int J Pediatr Otorhinolaryngol. 2013 Sep;77(9):1579-81. doi: 10.1016/j.ijporl.2013.07.014.

[115] Treatment with lavender aromatherapy in the post-anesthesia care unit reduces opioid requirements of morbidly obese patients undergoing laparoscopic adjustable gastric banding. Obes Surg. 2007 Jul;17(7):920-5. PMID: 17894152.

[116] Evaluation of aromatherapy in treating postoperative pain: pilot study. Pain Pract. 2006 Dec;6(4):273-7. DOI: 10.1111/j.1533-2500.2006.00095.x.

[117] Wound healing potential of lavender oil by acceleration of granulation and wound contraction through induction of TGF-Beta in a rat model. BMC Complement Altern Med. 2016; 16: 144. doi: 10.1186/s12906-016-1128-7.

[118] Hair Growth-Promoting Effects of Lavender Oil in C57BL/6 Mice. Toxicol Res. 2016 Apr; 32(2): 103–108. doi: 10.5487/TR.2016.32.2.103.

⚘CHAPTER 7

Month 4: Face The Facts

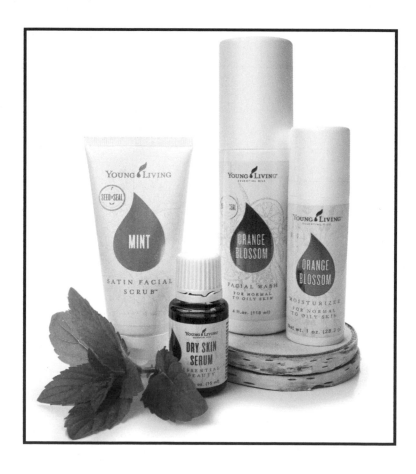

Your face is such an important part of your body. Not only does it contain important features like your eyes, nose, mouth, and ears, but its skin, together with the skin of your hands, is also one of the most exposed areas of your body. The human face has been of great interest to scientists because of the extraordinarily well-developed ability of humans to process, recognize, and extract information from the faces of others.[119] We know that attractive children and adults are judged more positively, even by those who know them, and exhibit more positive behaviors and traits than unattractive children and adults.[120]

Attractive people also appear to lead more favorable lives, pay lower bail amounts, and are more likely to be hired for jobs than less attractive individuals.[121,122] While the statement "beauty is in the eye of the beholder" is certainly true, it cannot be denied that the features of a face, including skin, play an important role in the way someone is perceived by others. It is also interesting to note that average faces and/or symmetrical faces are more attractive to others than distinctive and/or non-symmetrical faces.[123,124]

Another interesting fact about the face is that people will readily rate faces for perceived health and show very high agreement on such ratings.[125] Therefore, attractiveness judgements are likely to reflect judgements of apparent health. Other studies looked at how the features of facial skin, such as texture and color, influence the way individuals are judged. And as expected, it was shown that facial skin positively influenced attractiveness judgments.[126] These results underline the importance of the skin of your face and the importance of a good facial care program with good facial care products.

In the United States alone, the skin-care industry is a $43 billion per year business.[127] Healthy skin has a lot to do with self-esteem. Multiple studies have shown a higher incidence of clinical depression, anxiety disorder, and suicidal tendency among patients with common skin diseases. In fact, a large study conducted across 13 European countries evaluating the psychological burden of skin diseases found that clinical anxiety was present in 17.2%, suicidal ideation was reported by 12.7%, and clinical depression was present in 10.1% of patients with skin problems.[128]

Another study showed that skin was the first thing noticed about the face by 41% of the participants. Those with uneven facial skin texture were less likely to be perceived as attractive, confident, happy, healthy, and successful, as well as more likely to be judged as insecure and shy.[129] Research also shows that improving a physical trait such as the look of your facial skin improves attitude, personality, interpersonal interactions, and self-esteem.[130]

Orange Blossom Facial Wash

Get clearer skin by using Young Living's Orange Blossom Facial Wash. This gentle product was created with Lavender, Patchouli, Lemon, and Rosemary Essential Oils. Ingredients also include radish root ferment filtrate, olive fruit oil, cocoa seed butter, grapeseed oil, rose hips fruit oil, andiroba seed oil (also called crabwood seed oil), coconut oil, sunflower seed oil, vitamin E, microalgae oil, licorice root extract, camellia sinensis tea leaf extract, orange peel extract, lemon peel extract, apple fruit extract, sugarcane extract, English marigold flower extract, German chamomile flower extract, green algae extract, orange flower extract, St. John's-wort flower/leaf/stem extract, kelp extract, and rose flower extract.

Satin Facial Scrub

Polish and prep your skin with Young Living's naturally-derived Satin Facial Scrub. Made with apricot seed powder, it gently exfoliates the face to lift and remove dry, dead skin cells and reveal bright, even-looking skin. Use it to start the day or to take the day off; whenever you reach for it, you'll leave a clean, smooth slate for the next step in your skin care regimen. Young Living formulated this exfoliating scrub to bring you a natural way to cleanse your skin and reveal glowing, radiant skin.

With carefully selected ingredients, including mango butter and raspberry extract, you'll feel confident adding this gentle face exfoliator to your skin care routine, along with Young Living's other naturally derived personal care products. Plus, it has pure Peppermint Essential Oil for a minty scent and tingly fresh feel. Other ingredients include sunflower seed oil, apricot seed powder, pectin, mango seed butter, coconut oil, coco-glucoside, vitamin E, and raspberry fruit extract. Note: This product contains coconut ingredients.

Orange Blossom Moisturizer

Many people have to deal with facial skin dryness, which is induced by complex interactions between environmental and individual factors such as low environmental temperature, low humidity, chemical exposures, microorganisms, aging, psychological stress, and a variety of pathological skin conditions.[131] A daily moisturizing routine is a vital part of the management of people with dry skin. Significant improvements in skin health and quality can be observed when using a combination of mild cleansing, moisturizing, and sun protection.[132]

When used appropriately, skin cleansing and moisturizing products not only improve skin hydration by reducing water loss, but also help to restore the skin barrier and improve the aesthetic appearance of the face.[133] And because many facial skin products contain synthetic dyes and artificial fragrances, they can irritate and exacerbate unfavorable skin conditions. So, you should pay attention to the products used during your daily facial routine.

Treat your skin to a deep drink of hydration with Young Living's Orange Blossom Moisturizer, formulated specifically with essential oils for the skin. Made to benefit oily complexions, this moisturizer improves the appearance of skin without irritation from harsh chemicals. The Orange Blossom Moisturizer uses only naturally derived, plant-based ingredients that are vegan-friendly. It helps skin maintain optimal moisture balance, controls excess oil and shine, and preps your face for makeup with its natural-looking matte finish. This moisturizer is formulated without alcohol, parabens, phthalates, petrochemicals, animal-derived ingredients, synthetic preservatives, synthetic fragrances, or synthetic dyes. Note: This product contains coconut ingredients.

Young Living's Essential Beauty™ Serum (Dry)

Young Living's Essential Beauty™ Serum for dry skin contains essential oils like Blue Cypress and Lavender, which are known for their ability to restore the skin's natural moisture balance, and Cedarwood, Myrrh, Clove, and Royal Hawaiian Sandalwood™. Other ingredients include coconut oil, avocado oil, rosehip seed extract, jojoba seed oil, vitamin E, and wolfberry seed oil. Note: This product also contains soy and coconut/palm ingredients.

Note: None of the statements made about any of Young Living's products have been evaluated by the Food and Drug Administration. Young Living products are not intended to diagnose, treat, cure, or prevent any disease.

Most of the product information and text describing Young Living products is directly from Young Living Essential Oils, LC, and can be found online at youngliving.com

Sacred Sandalwood™, KidScents®, SniffleEase™, and Essential Beauty™ are trademarks of Young Living Essential Oils, LC.

Royal Hawaiian Sandalwood™ is a trademark of Jawmin, LLC.

Month 4 Shopping List:

Product Name	Item Number	PV
Orange Blossom Moisturizer	21622	33.5
Satin Facial Scrub - Mint	20454	16.75
Orange Blossom Facial Wash	20176	39.75
Essential Beauty™ Serum (Dry)	3782	20.75
	Total PV:	110.75
Bonus Essential Oil: Sacred Sandalwood™		
For Your Kiddo: SniffleEase™ Essential Oil		
Month 4 ER Points Earning Rate: 20%		
Rewards Points Earned this Month:		~22
Cumulative Reward Points:		~53

References:

[119] Facial attractiveness: evolutionary based research. Philos Trans R Soc Lond B Biol Sci. 2011 Jun 12; 366(1571): 1638–1659. doi: 10.1098/rstb.2010.0404.

[120] Maxims or myths of beauty? A meta-analytic and theoretical review. Psychol Bull. 2000 May;126(3):390-423. PMID: 10825783.

[121] Natural observations of the links between attractiveness and initial legal judgments. Pers. Soc. Psychol. B 17, 541–54710.1177/0146167291175009. doi:10.1177/0146167291175009.

[122] Gender and attractiveness biases in hiring decisions: are more experienced managers less biased? J. Appl. Psychol. 81, 11–2110.1037/0021-9010.81.1.11. doi:10.1037/0021-9010.81.1.11.

[123] The role of symmetry in attraction to average faces. Percept Psychophys. 2007 Nov;69(8):1273-7. PMID: 18078219.

[124] Symmetry, averageness, and feature size in the facial attractiveness of women. Acta Psychol (Amst). 2004 Nov;117(3):313-32. DOI: 10.1016/j.actpsy.2004.07.002.

[125] Facial symmetry and judgements of apparent health: support for a 'good genes' explanation of the attractiveness–symmetry relationship. Evol. Hum. Behav. 22, 417–42910.1016/S1090-5138(01)00083-6. doi:10.1016/S1090-5138(01)00083-6.

[126] When facial attractiveness is only skin deep. Perception. 2004;33(5):569-76. DOI: 10.1068/p3463.

[127] Skin care in the aging female: myths and truths. J Clin Invest. 2012 Feb 1; 122(2): 473–477. doi: 10.1172/JCI61978.

[128] The psychological burden of skin diseases: a cross-sectional multicenter study among dermatological out-patients in 13 European countries. J Invest Dermatol. 2015 Apr;135(4):984-991. doi: 10.1038/jid.2014.530.

[129] How People with Facial Acne Scars are Perceived in Society: an Online Survey. Dermatol Ther (Heidelb). 2016 Jun; 6(2): 207–218. doi: 10.1007/s13555-016-0113-x.

[130] Improving self-esteem by improving physical attractiveness. J Esthet Dent. 1997;9(1):44-6. PMID: 9468878.

[131] The Role of Moisturizers in Addressing Various Kinds of Dermatitis: A Review. Clin Med Res. 2017 Dec; 15(3-4): 75–87. doi: 10.3121/cmr.2017.1363.

[132] Cleansing, moisturizing, and sun-protection regimens for normal skin, self-perceived sensitive skin, and dermatologist-assessed sensitive skin. Dermatol Ther. 2004;17 Suppl 1:63-8. PMID: 14728701.

[133] Concepts in skin care maintenance. Cutis. 2005 Dec;76(6 Suppl):19-25. PMID: 16869178.

$\mathcal{L}$CHAPTER 8

Month 5: Gut Instinct

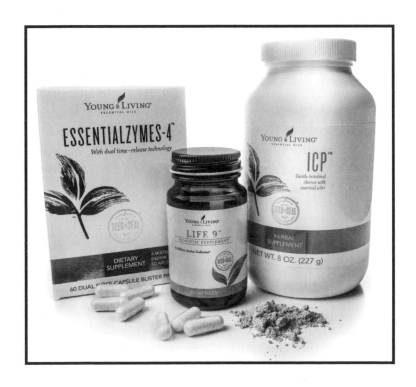

Re-read the title of this chapter: Gut Instinct! Do you listen and trust your gut? Do you sometimes have a sinking feeling in your stomach? Do you understand why the Persian poet Rumi said, "There is a voice that doesn't use words, listen to it"? Why is it that such expressions exist in so many cultures and languages? Well, let's dive into the gut and see.

If you have looked ahead at the chapter titles and topics, you may be wondering why I suggest to support your gut and your brain within two months of each other, since they are completely different organs and are not even closely located in the body. Historically, the gut has been seen as the main organ for food intake, breakdown, and absorption to supply our body with the necessary nutrients. At the same time the brain was seen as the command center, processing all incoming signals (sensory, visual, auditory, endocrine, and others) and then sending out commands to various parts of the body.

However, this traditional view of medical physiology has recently been challenged, and an entire new field of research has been developed: the research of the microbiome and its effect on other body systems, like the brain.[134] Today we know that the gut and brain are very closely linked. And a big reason for that is the microbiome.

What is the microbiome? By definition, it is the collective genome (genetic information) of all your micro-organisms such as bacteria, fungi, viruses, and archaea (bacteria-like organisms).[135] You harbor over 100 trillion of them, and most of these micro-organisms can be found in your gut, mainly in the colon.[136] But you will also find these microbes on the skin, on the scalp, in the vagina, in the nose and mouth, and possibly other places of the body such as the lungs, and even in previously considered sterile systems such as blood.[137] Bacteria from various microbiome systems interact extensively with each other within the human body.[138]

The microbiome has also been called "the last undiscovered human organ," highlighting the importance it has in human health.[139] Studies of the diversity of the human microbiome started as early as the 1680s when a researcher realized that the difference between oral and fecal bacteria was associated with different states of health or disease.[140]

It might be a little scary for you to hear this, but your microbiome cells outnumber your human cells by ten to one.[141] And if you look at the genetic information contained in the microbiome, the news gets even worse. It is estimated that 99% of the genetic information in a human body comes from the microbes, and only one percent is from the DNA obtained from your parents.[142] Researchers found that the microbiome contains 150 times more individual genes than human DNA, (3.3 million vs "only" 23,000 human genes).[143,144]

The diversity amongst the microbiome of individuals is immense: individuals are about 99.9% identical to one another in terms of genetic information contained in the DNA, but they can be 80-90% different from one another in terms of the genetic information contained in the microbiome of their gut and skin.[145]

It is time that we start to wonder what impact the use of chemicals in agriculture and in our households has on the microbiome of the soil.[146] The most frequently used herbicide and crop desiccant, and desecrator, is glyphosate. One of the glyphosate patents from 2010 states that it is an "antimicrobial agent," or in more basic terms, a very broad antibiotic with negative effects on growth of bacteria and other types of micro-organisms. [147]

Since 1974, over 1.6 billion kilograms of the glyphosate active ingredient have been put on the fields in the U.S. alone, and about five to six times more has been used internationally (8.6 billion kilograms). Globally, its use has risen almost 15-fold since so-called genetically engineered glyphosate-tolerant crops were introduced in 1996.[148]

The effects of an antibiotic are not only disastrous for the microbiome of the soil but also for the hugely important microbiome in our gut.[149,150] Even doses previously considered as safe have shown to change the microbiome.[151] Negative changes in the human microbiome cause emotional, mental, and developmental issues, as well as obesity and other significant health problems. Several studies have shown the negative effects glyphosate has on the microbiome, leading to complications in other organs such as the brain.[152]

It is also interesting that body weight, and therefore whether you are obese or not, might be decided to a large extent by the "bugs" in your gut.[153,154,155] Fecal transplants using bacteria from the feces of obese mice, relocated into lean mice, caused the lean mice to become obese and vice versa.[156,157,158] In fact, fecal transplants date back as early as the fourth century in China, where "Yellow Soup" was used to treat severe food poisoning and diarrhea.[159] In recent years, over 700 patients have been treated with such transplants for a variety of health conditions, many with resounding success.[160]

A healthy microbiome is crucial for human health.[161,162] The microbiome is certainly important for gut health.[163] However, it has far more reaching effects on the human body. We now know that the microbes in your gut have significant influence on a variety of illnesses such as autoimmune,[164,165] cardiovascular,[166] respiratory,[167] and infectious diseases,[168] mental sicknesses including Alzheimer's Disease,[169,170,171,172] and obesity,[173] just to name a few. Equipped with this knowledge about the microbiome and the information about endocrine disruptors and their catastrophic effects on human health and the environment, we need to search for healthier food alternatives. We should use our Gut Instinct!

But how do we connect the gut and the brain, and why was the gut called "the second brain" for thousands of years? Is it surprising that the bugs in your gut can influence your emotions, mood, thinking, cognition, memory, and much more?[174,175,176] How does this possibly work? Well, if the microbiome in your gut is not well-balanced and gets inflamed, then specific reactions in the bacteria, the gut itself, and the gut wall will release inflammatory compounds (via the activation of parts of our immune system)[177] which will then get into the bloodstream and reach the brain and all other organ systems.[178,179] In addition, the cells of the gut will send signals through the vagal nerve as well as through hormones (endocrine system) to the brain and cause inflammation there.[180]

It is now known that important brain structures, like the hippocampus in the limbic system, are partially responsible for your memory, emotions, spatial awareness, and more, and will suffer quickly from brain inflammation.[181] As a result, your hippocampus will shrink in size, which will cause your memory abilities to decrease and your emotions to go haywire.[182] Both aspects of the unhealthy Western diet (lower intakes of nutrient-dense foods and higher intakes of unhealthy foods) are each independently associated with smaller left hippocampal volume.[183]

Now for the great news: you can significantly influence your microbiome and regrow parts of your brain like the hippocampus.[184] Your lifestyle, consumption of prebiotics (fibers) and probiotics (beneficial bacteria), and an overall healthy balanced food intake have shown to make a huge difference in the development, and even reversal, of certain brain conditions.[185,186] Physical exercise and cardiovascular fitness have also been shown to directly influence the quality and diversity of your microbiome and therefore to improve healthy brain function.[187,188] And the intake of probiotics had a great influence on the stability of emotional memory and emotional decision-making,[189] all functions which involve the hippocampus.

Hopefully, you now understand the importance of chemical-free organic agriculture and the effects that those pesticides can have on the microbiome of the soil and the microbiome in your own body. Young Living products offer you a lifestyle that enables you to decrease the amount of environmental poisons contaminating the food chain, while directly decreasing the amount of harsh chemicals reaching your cells and your microbiome. In addition, you can promote a healthy microbiome by using healthy products such as the probiotic blend Life 9™ (or KidScents® MightyPro™ for your children) and those containing healthy fibers such as ICP™ and NingXia Red®.

Please understand that you completely depend on a healthy microbiome in your gut and on your skin. Do not adversely affect it with bad nutrition, a sedentary lifestyle, and the harsh toxic chemicals found in commercial household cleaners, detergents, antibacterial soaps, and makeup. Love and support your bugs and they will love and support you!

According to the WHO and the Food and Agricultural Organization of the United Nations, probiotics are defined as "living micro-organisms, which when administered in adequate amounts confer health benefits on the host."[190] They work through a variety of mechanisms including suppressing bad bacteria,[191] competing with receptor sites within the gut lining cells,[192] modulating the intestinal immunity,[193] stabilizing the microbiome,[194] and affecting the composition and function of the microbiome.[195]

Probiotics are now being proposed as a preventive and therapeutic way to improve wellness and health. They are being classified as "functional food" or "functional drinks." Probiotics are now also added to skin care products, establishing the "functional skin care" category, as well as to agricultural soil-improving products, creating the field of "functional agriculture." Probiotics have shown to be beneficial for a variety of conditions such as cardiovascular diseases,[196,197] metabolic syndromes and obesity,[198,199] immune disorders including auto-immune diseases,[200] neurological diseases including Alzheimer's disease,[201,202,203] diabetes,[204,205] and more.

The term "probiotic" covers a wide variety of beneficial bacterial families, so it cannot be concluded that just because one particular blend was used in one study that it will benefit patients with other conditions. It should also be noted that the claims allowed in connection with the term "probiotics" vary tremendously depending on the region in which you live. But large international organizations such as the WHO have adopted significant language such as "Probiotic benefits include physical, mental, and social wellbeing. [They] can be either administered orally or topically."[206]

Life 9™

Young Living's Life 9™ is a proprietary, high-potency probiotic supplement, formulated with nine different strains or families of probiotic bacteria including Lactobacillus acidophilus, Bifidobacterium lactis, Lactobacillus plantarum, Lactobacillus rhamnosus, Lactobacillus salivarius, Streptococcus thermophilus, Bifidobacterium breve, Bifidobacterium bifidum, and Bifidobacterium longum. Each capsule contains a whopping 17 billion live cultures. Life 9™ is specially designed with delayed-release capsules, a dual-sorbent desiccant, and a specific bottle and cap that ensure your Life 9™ stays fresh and effective. This product promotes healthy digestion, supports gut health, and helps maintain normal intestinal function for overall support of a healthy immune system.

Prebiotics are just as important as probiotics.[207] What are prebiotics? They are fibers used by the gut bacteria as food. Humans are not able to digest all types of fiber. However, the bacteria from the microbiome in the gut will use those fibers (complex carbohydrates and plant polysaccharides) as an energy source.[208] The intake of such prebiotic fibers has shown to quickly improve the diversity and richness of the human gastrointestinal microbiome.[209] Human studies from around the globe reveal that greater dietary fiber intake is associated with increased gastrointestinal microbial community diversity.[210]

ICP™

Young Living's ICP™ provides ingredients such as psyllium, oat bran, and flax and fennel seeds to form a combination of soluble and insoluble fibers. Enhanced with a special blend of essential oils, the fibers work to decrease the buildup of waste, improve nutrient absorption, and help maintain a healthy heart. ICP™ provides two grams of dietary fiber, one gram of soluble fiber, and one gram of insoluble fiber per serving. This supplement includes Fennel, Anise, Tarragon, Ginger, Lemongrass, and Rosemary Essential Oils.

Many people ask me if essential oils have a negative impact on the microbiome or on the intake of probiotics. There are a handful of studies discussing this question. These studies show that essential oils had either no effect at all on the microbiome[211] or that they even benefited the microbiome and the probiotics in the sense that they decreased the number of pathological bacteria in the gut while leaving the beneficial ones alone or even by increasing the number of good bacteria![212,213,214,215,216,217,218]

Essentialzymes-4™

A variety of digestive enzymes are produced by the body to aid in the digestion of food. Enzyme supplementation may provide reliable help in conditions with low enzyme levels characterized by an impairment of digestive function.[219] Essentialzymes-4™ is a multi-spectrum enzyme complex specially formulated to aid the critically needed digestion of dietary fats, proteins, fiber, and carbohydrates commonly found in the modern processed diet. The dual time-release technology releases the animal- and plant-based enzymes at separate times within the digestive tract, allowing for optimal nutrient absorption. The first capsule contains important enzymes such as amylase, lipase, cellulase, peptidase, phytase, bromelain, and papain mixed with Anise, Ginger, Rosemary, Tarragon, and Fennel Essential Oils. The second capsule contains bee pollen powder, pancreatin, and lipase mixed with Ginger, Fennel, Tarragon, Anise, and Lemongrass Essential Oils.

Now you know about the importance of the microbiome and how to support it with great, natural products. It is time to love and support your gut.

Bonus Product: ComforTone®

Irregular bowel movements occur commonly among people today. As a physician, I prefer my patients to have one to two bowel movements daily. If this seems impossible for you, don't worry. Several herbs can treat conditions with slow bowel movements.

ComforTone® provides a combination of natural herbs and essential oils that may support digestive health and wellness. Key ingredients are cascara sagrada bark, barberry bark, burdock root, psyllium seeds, garlic, apple pectin, licorice root, fennel seeds, ginger root, as well as Tarragon, Ginger, Tangerine, Rosemary, Anise, Peppermint, Ocotea, and German Chamomile Essential Oils. This product should quickly show results. It is not intended for long-term use.

Note: None of the statements made about any of Young Living's products have been evaluated by the Food and Drug Administration. Young Living products are not intended to diagnose, treat, cure, or prevent any disease.

AromaEase™, KidScents®, MightyPro™, Life 9™, ICP™, Essentialzymes-4™, and ComforTone® are trademarks of Young Living Essential Oils, LC.

Month 5 Shopping List:

Product Name	Item Number	PV
Life 9™	18299	29.5
ICP™	3208	26.5
Essentialzymes-4™	4645	51.25
	Total PV:	107.25
Bonus Essential Oil: AromaEase™		
For Your Kiddo: MightyPro™		
Month 5 ER Points Earning Rate: 20%		
Rewards Points Earned this Month:		~22
Cumulative Reward Points:		~74

References:

[134] The gut microbiome in health and in disease. Curr Opin Gastroenterol. 2015 Jan; 31(1): 69–75. doi: 10.1097/MOG.0000000000000139.

[135] Defining the Human Microbiome. Nutr Rev. 2012 Aug; 70(Suppl 1): S38–S44. doi: 10.1111/j.1753-4887.2012.00493.x.

[136] The human microbiome project. Nature. 2007 Oct 18;449(7164):804-10. DOI: 10.1038/nature06244.

[137] Involvement of gut microbiome in human health and disease: brief overview, knowledge gaps and research opportunities. Gut Pathog. 2018; 10: 3. doi: 10.1186/s13099-018-0230-4.

[138] Microbial co-occurrence relationships in the human microbiome. PLoS Comput Biol. 2012;8(7):e1002606. doi: 10.1371/journal.pcbi.1002606.

[139] The microbiome as a human organ. Clin Microbiol Infect. 2012 Jul;18 Suppl 4:2-4. doi: 10.1111/j.1469-0691.2012.03916.x.

[140] An abstract of a Letter from Antonie van Leeuwenhoek, Sep. 12, 1683. About Animals in the scrurf of the Teeth. Philosophical Transactions of the Royal Society of London. 1684;14:568–574.

[141] NIH Human Microbiome Project defines normal bacterial makeup of the body. https://www.nih.gov/news-events/news-releases/nih-human-microbiome-project-defines-normal-bacterial-makeup-body.

[142] Metagenomic Analysis of the Human Distal Gut Microbiome. Science. 2006 Jun 2; 312(5778): 1355–1359. doi: 10.1126/science.1124234.

[143] A human gut microbial gene catalogue established by metagenomic sequencing. Nature volume 464, 2010: pages 59–65.

[144] Finishing the euchromatic sequence of the human genome. Nature. 2004 Oct 21;431(7011):931-45. DOI: 10.1038/nature03001.

[145] Defining the Human Microbiome. Nutr Rev. 2012 Aug; 70(Suppl 1): S38–S44. doi: 10.1111/j.1753-4887.2012.00493.x.

[146] Measuring the effects of pesticides on bacterial communities in soil: A critical review. European Journal of Soil Biology. Volume 49, March–April 2012, Pages 22-30.

[147] Glyphosate formulations and their use for the inhibition of 5-enolpyruvylshikimate-3-phosphate synthase. Google Patents. https://patents.google.com/patent/US7771736B2/en.

[148] Trends in glyphosate herbicide use in the United States and globally. Environ Sci Eur. 2016; 28(1): 3. doi: 10.1186/s12302-016-0070-0.

[149] Glyphosate-Induced Specific and Widespread Perturbations in the Metabolome of Soil Pseudomonas Species. Front. Environ. Sci., 20 June 2017.

[150] The pervasive effects of an antibiotic on the human gut microbiota, as revealed by deep 16S rRNA sequencing. PLoS Biol. 2008 Nov 18;6(11):e280. doi: 10.1371/journal.pbio.0060280.

[151] The Ramazzini Institute 13-week pilot study on glyphosate and Roundup administered at human-equivalent dose to Sprague Dawley rats: effects on the microbiome. Environ Health. 2018 May 29;17(1):50. doi: 10.1186/s12940-018-0394-x.

[152] Glyphosate based- herbicide exposure affects gut microbiota, anxiety and depression-like behaviors in mice. Neurotoxicol Teratol. 2018 May - Jun;67:44-49. doi: 10.1016/j.ntt.2018.04.002.

[153] A core gut microbiome in obese and lean twins. Nature. 2009 Jan 22;457(7228):480-4. doi: 10.1038/nature07540.

[154] Microbiota from the distal guts of lean and obese adolescents exhibit

partial functional redundancy besides clear differences in community structure. Environ Microbiol. 2013 Jan;15(1):211-26. doi: 10.1111/j.1462-2920.2012.02845.x.

[155] The relationship between gut microbiota and weight gain in humans. Future Microbiol. 2012 Jan;7(1):91-109. doi: 10.2217/fmb.11.142.

[156] Obesity, metabolic syndrome, and microbiota: multiple interactions. J Clin Gastroenterol. 2010 Sep;44 Suppl 1:S16-8. doi: 10.1097/MCG.0b013e3181dd8b64.

[157] Gut microbiota and obesity: implications for fecal microbiota transplantation therapy. Hormones (Athens). 2017 Jul;16(3):223-234. doi: 10.14310/horm.2002.1742.

[158] Treating Obesity and Metabolic Syndrome with Fecal Microbiota Transplantation. Yale J Biol Med. 2016 Sep 30;89(3):383-388. PMID: 27698622.

[159] Should we standardize the 1,700-year-old fecal microbiota transplantation? Am J Gastroenterol. 2012 Nov;107(11):1755; author reply p.1755-6. doi: 10.1038/ajg.2012.251.

[160] Fecal microbiota transplantation in metabolic syndrome: History, present and future. Gut Microbes. 2017; 8(3): 253–267. doi: 10.1080/19490976.2017.1293224.

[161] Rapidly expanding knowledge on the role of the gut microbiome in health and disease. Biochim Biophys Acta. 2014 Oct;1842(10):1981-1992. doi: 10.1016/j.bbadis.2014.05.023.

[162] The potential impact of gut microbiota on your health:Current status and future challenges. Asian Pac J Allergy Immunol. 2016 Dec;34(4):249-264. doi: 10.12932/AP0803.

[163] The Intestinal Microbiota in Health and Disease. Curr Opin Gastroenterol. 2012 Jan; 28(1): 63–69. doi: 10.1097/MOG.0b013e32834d61e9.

[164] Clinical Evidence for the Microbiome in Inflammatory Diseases. Front Immunol. 2017; 8: 400. doi: 10.3389/fimmu.2017.00400.

[165] Diet, microbiota and autoimmune diseases. Lupus. 2014 May;23(6):518-26. doi: 10.1177/0961203313501401.

[166] The gut microbiome in atherosclerotic cardiovascular disease. Nat Commun. 2017; 8: 845. doi: 10.1038/s41467-017-00900-1.

[167] Early-Life Intestine Microbiota and Lung Health in Children. J Immunol Res. 2017; 2017: 8450496. doi: 10.1155/2017/8450496.

[168] The Intestinal Microbiome in Infectious Diseases: The Clinical Relevance of a Rapidly Emerging Field. Open Forum Infect Dis. 2017 Summer; 4(3): ofx144. doi: 10.1093/ofid/ofx144.

[169] Gut microbiota's effect on mental health: The gut-brain axis. Clin Pract. 2017 Sep 15; 7(4): 987. doi: 10.4081/cp.2017.987.

[170] A randomized controlled trial to test the effect of multispecies probiotics on cognitive reactivity to sad mood. Brain Behav Immun. 2015 Aug;48:258-64. doi: 10.1016/j.bbi.2015.04.003.

Month 5: Gut Instinct

[171] Influence of gut microbiota on neuropsychiatric disorders. World J Gastroenterol. 2017 Aug 14; 23(30): 5486–5498. doi: 10.3748/wjg.v23. i30.5486.

[172] The Gut Microbiota and Alzheimer's Disease. J Alzheimers Dis. 2017;58(1):1-15. doi: 10.3233/JAD-161141.

[173] The Gut Microbiome and Its Role in Obesity. Nutr Today. 2016 Jul-Aug; 51(4): 167–174. doi: 10.1097/NT.0000000000000167.

[174] The Gut Microbiome and the Brain. J Med Food. 2014 Dec 1; 17(12): 1261–1272. doi: 10.1089/jmf.2014.7000.

[175] Gut/brain axis and the microbiota. J Clin Invest. 2015 Mar 2;125(3):926-38. doi: 10.1172/JCI76304.

[176] Gut microbes and the brain: paradigm shift in neuroscience. J Neurosci. 2014 Nov 12;34(46):15490-6. doi: 10.1523/JNEUROSCI.3299-14.2014.

[177] Immune-Microbiota Interactions: Dysbiosis as a Global Health Issue. Curr Allergy Asthma Rep. 2016 Feb;16(2):13. doi: 10.1007/s11882-015-0590-5.

[178] The role of the gut microbiome in systemic inflammatory disease. BMJ. 2018 Jan 8;360:j5145. doi: 10.1136/bmj.j5145.

[179] Linking the Human Gut Microbiome to Inflammatory Cytokine Production Capacity. Cell. 2016 Nov 3; 167(4): 1125–1136.e8. doi: 10.1016/j. cell.2016.10.020.

[180] The Gut Microbiome Feelings of the Brain: A Perspective for Non-Microbiologists. Microorganisms. 2017 Dec; 5(4): 66. doi: 10.3390/microorganisms5040066.

[181] Chronic brain inflammation leads to a decline in hippocampal NMDA-R1 receptors. J Neuroinflammation. 2004; 1: 12. doi: 10.1186/1742-2094-1-12.

[182] Gut to Brain Dysbiosis: Mechanisms Linking Western Diet Consumption, the Microbiome, and Cognitive Impairment. Front Behav Neurosci. 2017; 11: 9. doi: 10.3389/fnbeh.2017.00009.

[183] Western diet is associated with a smaller hippocampus: a longitudinal investigation. BMC Med. 2015 Sep 8;13:215. doi: 10.1186/s12916-015-0461-x.

[184] Adult Hippocampal Neurogenesis Is Regulated by the Microbiome. Biol Psychiatry. 2015 Aug 15;78(4):e7-9. doi: 10.1016/j.biopsych.2014.12.023.

[185] Modulation of Gut Microbiota-Brain Axis by Probiotics, Prebiotics, and Diet. J Agric Food Chem. 2015 Sep 16;63(36):7885-95. doi: 10.1021/acs. jafc.5b02404.

[186] Stress and adolescent hippocampal neurogenesis: diet and exercise as cognitive modulators. Transl Psychiatry. 2017 Apr; 7(4): e1081. doi: 10.1038/tp.2017.48.

[187] The effects of hormones and physical exercise on hippocampal structural plasticity. Front Neuroendocrinol. 2016 Apr;41:23-43. doi: 10.1016/j. yfrne.2016.03.001.

[188] Exercise Modifies the Gut Microbiota with Positive Health Effects. Oxid Med Cell Longev. 2017; 2017: 3831972. doi: 10.1155/2017/3831972.

[189] Probiotics drive gut microbiome triggering emotional brain signatures. Gut Microbes. 2018 May 3:1-11. doi: 10.1080/19490976.2018.1460015.

[190] Joint FAO/WHO Expert Consultation on Evaluation of Health and Nutritional Properties of Probiotics in Food Including Powder Milk with Live Lactic Acid Bacteria, and Joint FAO/WHO Working Group on Drafting Guidelines for the Evaluation of Probiotics in Food (2006) Probiotics in food: health and nutritional properties and guidelines for evaluation. http://www.fao.org/3/a-a0512e.pdf.

[191] Human-derived probiotic Lactobacillus reuteri demonstrate antimicrobial activities targeting diverse enteric bacterial pathogens. Anaerobe. 2008 Jun;14(3):166-71. doi: 10.1016/j.anaerobe.2008.02.001.

[192] Role of commercial probiotic strains against human pathogen adhesion to intestinal mucus. Lett Appl Microbiol. 2007 Oct;45(4):454-60. DOI: 10.1111/j.1472-765X.2007.02212.x.

[193] Probiotics-host communication: Modulation of signaling pathways in the intestine. Gut Microbes. 2010 May-Jun;1(3):148-63. PMID: 20672012.

[194] The effect of a multispecies probiotic mixture on the symptoms and fecal microbiota in diarrhea-dominant irritable bowel syndrome: a randomized, double-blind, placebo-controlled trial. J Clin Gastroenterol. 2012 Mar;46(3):220-7. doi: 10.1097/MCG.0b013e31823712b1.

[195] Effects of probiotics on gut microbiota: mechanisms of intestinal immunomodulation and neuromodulation. Therap Adv Gastroenterol. 2013 Jan; 6(1): 39–51. doi: 10.1177/1756283X12459294.

[196] The influence of the human microbiome and probiotics on cardiovascular health. Gut Microbes. 2014;5(6):719-28. doi: 10.4161/19490976.2014.983775.

[197] 'The way to a man's heart is through his gut microbiota'--dietary pro- and prebiotics for the management of cardiovascular risk. Proc Nutr Soc. 2014 May;73(2):172-85. doi: 10.1017/S0029665113003911.

[198] Gut microbiome and metabolic diseases. Semin Immunopathol. 2014 Jan;36(1):103-14. doi: 10.1007/s00281-013-0399-z.

[199] The development of probiotic treatment in obesity: a review. Benef Microbes. 2014 Mar;5(1):19-28. doi: 10.3920/BM2012.0069.

[200] A probiotic modulates the microbiome and immunity in multiple sclerosis. Ann Neurol. 2018 Jun;83(6):1147-1161. doi: 10.1002/ana.25244.

[201] Microbiota modulation counteracts Alzheimer's disease progression influencing neuronal proteolysis and gut hormones plasma levels. Sci Rep. 2017; 7: 2426. doi: 10.1038/s41598-017-02587-2.

[202] Alzheimer's disease and the microbiome. Front Cell Neurosci. 2013; 7: 153. doi: 10.3389/fncel.2013.00153.

[203] Effect of Probiotic Supplementation on Cognitive Function and Metabolic Status in Alzheimer's Disease: A Randomized, Double-Blind and Controlled Trial. Front Aging Neurosci. 2016; 8: 256. doi: 10.3389/fnagi.2016.00256.

[204] The Future of Diabetes Management by Healthy Probiotic Microorganisms. Curr Diabetes Rev. 2017;13(6):582-589. doi: 10.2174/1573

399812666161014112515.

[205] Effects of probiotic supplementation on glycaemic control and lipid profiles in gestational diabetes: A randomized, double-blind, placebo-controlled trial. Diabetes Metab. 2016 Sep;42(4):234-41. doi: 10.1016/j.diabet.2016.04.009.

[206] Guidelines for the Evaluation of Probiotics in Food. Report of a Joint FAO/ WHO Working Group on Drafting Guidelines for the Evaluation of Probiotics in Food. www.who.int/foodsafety/fs_management/en/probiotic_guidelines. pdf.

[207] Dietary fiber and prebiotics and the gastrointestinal microbiota. Gut Microbes. 2017; 8(2): 172–184. doi: 10.1080/19490976.2017.1290756.

[208] Fiber and prebiotics: mechanisms and health benefits. Nutrients. 2013 Apr 22;5(4):1417-35. doi: 10.3390/nu5041417.

[209] Diet rapidly and reproducibly alters the human gut microbiome. Nature. 2014 Jan 23;505(7484):559-63. doi: 10.1038/nature12820.

[210] Gut Microbiome: Westernization and the Disappearance of Intestinal Diversity. Curr Biol. 2015 Jul 20;25(14):R611-3. doi: 10.1016/j. cub.2015.05.040.

[211] The effect of herbs and their associated essential oils on performance, dietary digestibility and gut microflora in chickens from 7 to 28 days of age. Br Poult Sci. 2007 Aug;48(4):496-506. PMID: 17701503.

[212] Development of Probiotic Candidate in Combination with Essential Oils from Medicinal Plant and Their Effect on Enteric Pathogens: A Review. Gastroenterol Res Pract. 2012; 2012: 457150. doi: 10.1155/2012/457150.

[213] Essential oils have different effects on human pathogenic and commensal bacteria in mixed faecal fermentations compared with pure cultures. Microbiology. 2015 Feb;161(Pt 2):441-9. doi: 10.1099/mic.0.000009.

[214] Essential oils in the treatment of intestinal dysbiosis: A preliminary in vitro study. Altern Med Rev. 2009 Dec;14(4):380-4. PMID: 20030464.

[215] The treatment of small intestinal bacterial overgrowth with enteric-coated peppermint oil: a case report. Altern Med Rev. 2002 Oct;7(5):410-7. PMID: 12410625.

[216] Comparison of the antibacterial activity of essential oils and extracts of medicinal and culinary herbs to investigate potential new treatments for irritable bowel syndrome. BMC Complement Altern Med. 2013 Nov 28;13:338. doi: 10.1186/1472-6882-13-338..

[217] Intestinal Microbiome-Metabolome Responses to Essential Oils in Piglets. Front Microbiol. 2018; 9: 1988. doi: 10.3389/fmicb.2018.01988.

[218] Oregano Essential Oil Improves Intestinal Morphology and Expression of Tight Junction Proteins Associated with Modulation of Selected Intestinal Bacteria and Immune Status in a Pig Model. Biomed Res Int. 2016; 2016: 5436738. doi: 10.1155/2016/5436738.

[219] Digestive Enzyme Supplementation in Gastrointestinal Diseases. Curr Drug Metab. 2016 Feb; 17(2): 187–193. doi: 10.2174/13892002170216011 4150137.

❧CHAPTER 9

Month 6: Mind Your Health

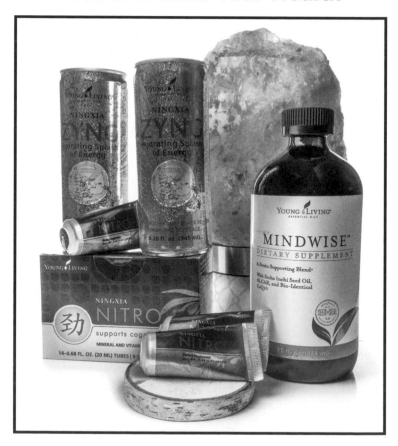

Health is partially a state of mind. If your brain does not function properly, it will be very difficult to adapt to a healthy lifestyle. Memory, mood stability, cognitive function, sleep, and many brain processes are vital for a happy life. According to the World Health Organization, mental health disorders are one of the leading causes of disability worldwide.[220] The WHO also stated recently that the burden of mental disorders continues to grow, with significant impacts on health, major social and human rights, and economies in all countries of the world.[221]

The Global Burden of Disease 2010 Study estimated that neurologic conditions, including dementia and Alzheimer's, were the third leading cause of "years lived with disability."[222] The occurrence of dementia, particularly Alzheimer's Disease, is increasing fast in both developing and developed countries.[223] For men between the ages of 60 and 90, the incidence of dementia increases by two times and the prevalence increase is 55.25-fold compared to men below 60. For women in that same age range, the incidence increases by 41 times while the prevalence increase is 77-fold compared to women below 60.[224] Incidence describes how many new cases occur in a given time and is therefore an indicator of risk, whereas prevalence means the proportion of cases in the population at a given time.

Of course, older people are not the only ones who suffer from mental health issues. Developmental disorders, including autism in children and young adults, are also increasing dramatically. Approximately one in every four to five young adults in the U.S. today meets the criteria for a mental disorder with severe impairment across their lifetime.[225]

Overall, there is no doubt that neurological/mental diseases are on a steep incline. This is astonishing considering how simple and cheap the prevention of many of these cases could be. It all has to do with an active and healthy lifestyle and the microbiome. It is now known that alterations in the gut microbiome may play a pathophysiological role in human brain diseases, including autism spectrum disorder, anxiety, depression, and chronic pain.[226] This knowledge opens new doors for the prevention and treatment of mental diseases by influencing the bugs in the gut. Probiotics are now also being called "psychobiotics" to highlight their potential for use in offsetting or preventing neurological disorders.[227]

As we get older, our birthdays are celebrated with "over the hill" and similar expressions indicating that at a certain age we have reached our peak and are now going down. We've also been told that learning is only for young people. But recently, many resources have been invested in research to study neuroplasticity, which is the capability of the brain to rewire itself and improve its own function.

Studies showed that even while aging, the brain has the capacity to increase neural activity and develop better cognitive function, as proven by increased brain tissue volumes in certain areas of the brain.[228] Today it is generally accepted that the adult brain is far from static.[229] Neuroplasticity has no age limit! We also know that neuroplasticity can easily be boosted by exercise.[230,231] So, what are you waiting for? Get moving. Are you too tired? Need an energy shot?

In today's society, many people try to overcome mental and physical fatigue by consuming so-called "energy" drinks. Low energy, fatigue, restless sleep, stress, and hormone disturbances are hallmarks of our time. Consumers are looking for a quick solution, and energy drink consumption is growing rapidly within the United States and worldwide.[232] The extreme reliance on these drinks represents a global public health problem, especially among adolescents and young adults.[233]

Caffeine use is increasing worldwide, because people are looking to boost their concentration and memory enhancement as well as improve physical performance.[234] However, reports of caffeine toxicity from energy drink consumption are increasing. Their potentially severe adverse effects include cardiovascular problems,[235,236] blood sugar regulation and diabetes,[237] obesity,[238] non-alcoholic liver disease, musculoskeletal problems, neurological problems,[239] dental erosion, renal complications, and increase in alcohol consumption when mixed into alcoholic beverages.[240]

One analysis showed that the incidence of moderate to major adverse effects of energy drink-related toxicity was 15.2% and 39.3% for non-alcoholic and alcoholic energy drinks, respectively. Major adverse effects included seizures, heart arrhythmias, and tachypnea (abnormally rapid breathing).[241] Unfortunately, there is emerging evidence of high-risk consumption patterns and acute poisoning.

One study showed that 87% of consumers drinking recreational energy drinks reported symptoms like palpitations, agitation, tremors, and gastrointestinal issues.[242] About half of them required hospitalization. Emergency room visits related to energy drink consumption doubled in four years.[243] Medical societies and public health institutions have been calling for better controls to protect consumers, especially our youth.[244,245]

Young Living created a series of great essential oil-based products like NingXia Nitro™, NingXia Zyng™, and Ningxia Red® to support healthy energy levels and replace commercially-available and potentially very dangerous "energy drinks." Instead of loading their products with high doses of caffeine, sugars, or simple sugar-analogs, Young Living blended natural extracts and pulp from healthy fruits with other plants, and added essential oils to achieve the same (or better) effects in a natural, non-harming way.

The very modest caffeine contents in NingXia Nitro™ and NingXia Zyng™ come from natural sources such as green tea, yerba mate, or chocolate essential oil. These products contain little sugar and are low-glycemic index drinks. They represent a true healthy alternative to the dangerous energy drinks sold in stores. In addition, the ingredients in NingXia Zyng™ and NingXia Nitro™ include some of the many essential oils made from spices, fruits, or plants that have shown to support healthy brain function.[246, 247,248,249,250,251]

NingXia Nitro™

NingXia Nitro™ is Young Living's healthy energy and cognitive function enhancer. It supports alertness as well as mental and physical fitness. With NingXia Nitro™, you'll get a quick pick-me-up without the sugar or caffeine overload. NingXia Nitro™ is infused with essential oils, botanical extracts, D-ribose, Korean ginseng, and green tea extract. D-ribose has shown to reduce jitteriness during and after caffeine consumption[252] while itself it is an excellent ATP/energy booster. Adenosine triphosphate (ATP) is the energy currency of the body. Green tea has long been known to improve performance. One study even showed a 24% boost of exercise endurance.[253]

NingXia Nitro™ also includes Vanilla, Chocolate, Yerba Mate, Spearmint, Peppermint, Nutmeg, and Black Pepper Essential Oils, as well as wolfberry seed oil. Who would have guessed that these little tubes could hold so much power? It's time to ditch the common caffeine and sugar-loaded energy drinks and switch to a healthy alternative. Keep a few NingXia Nitro™ tubes on hand to help you stay sharp throughout the workday, or energized while caring for your kiddos, or for an extra boost during your workout.

NingXia Zyng™

NingXia Zyng™ is a hydrating splash of essential oil-infused goodness. It was created by Young Living to offer a refreshing, slightly carbonated drink for a quick lift-me-up. It contains the same whole-fruit Ningxia wolfberry puree found in the popular superfruit supplement, NingXia Red®, as well as sparkling water, pear and blackberry juices, and a hint of Lime and Black Pepper Essential Oils. With natural flavors and sweeteners, white tea extract, and added vitamins, NingXia Zyng™ delivers 35mg of naturally occurring caffeine and only 35 calories per can, making it a sweet, guilt-free boost for your entire day. NingXia Zyng™ is a great alternative for those loved ones who are addicted to soda.

MindWise™

Brain health also depends on proper levels of fats essential for brain function. Omega-3 fatty acids are known to be very important for a healthy brain and enhanced cognitive function.[254] The brain is normally rich in omega-3 long-chain polyunsaturated fatty acid (PUFA). These fatty acids act as structural components of nerves and brain cells including their membranes, thereby influencing brain function. An adequate intake of omega-3 PUFA is essential for optimal visual function and neural development.[255] These fatty acids are also important for cardiovascular health.

Dietary supplementation with omega-3 fatty acids significantly reduced the risk of overall cardiovascular deaths, sudden cardiac death, and nonfatal cardiovascular events such as heart attacks and strokes.[256] PUFA consumption lowers plasma triglycerides, resting heart rate, and blood pressure while improving heart function, lowering inflammation, decreasing arrhythmia (irregular heart beat), and improving vascular (blood vessel) function.[257] Omega-3 fatty acids include alpha-linolenic acid

(ALA), eicosapentaenoic acid (EPA), docosahexaenoic acid (DHA), and their metabolites. These can be found in foods: Flaxseed is rich in ALA, nuts and fish are rich in EPA, and fish is rich in DHA.

In the body, ALA is converted to DHA and EPA. DHA is the principal omega-3 fatty acid in the gray matter, where brain processing takes place. The importance of DHA intake has been reported for patients with a variety of brain disorders such as major depressive and bipolar disorders, Alzheimer's disease, Parkinson's disease, and other disorders.[258]

Another type of fat called medium-chained triglycerides (MCTs) is also very important for proper brain function. Studies showed that medium-chain triglyceride ingestion significantly improves cognition.[259,260,261] Other compounds such as co-enzyme Q10 are very important for the brain,[262] heart, and muscles. Acetyl-l-carnitine (ALCAR) has shown in studies to prevent age-related mitochondrial dysfunction and to exert neuroprotective effects.[263] Glycerylphosphorylcholine (GPC) also supports healthy mitochondrial function in the brain and other cells of the body.[264]

Vitamin D is involved in many processes of our body. We know that when it comes to the brain, vitamin D receptors are widespread in brain tissue, and vitamin D displays neuro-protective effects including the clearance of amyloid plaques, a hallmark of Alzheimer's disease.[265] For example, the relative risk of cognitive decline was 60% higher in elderly adults with severely deficient Vitamin D levels when compared with those with sufficient levels[266].

We also know that several essential oils and other extracts from plants have major beneficial effects on brain health. One study described that essential oils and their components from Nigella sativa (fennel), Acorus gramineus (Japanese sweet flag), Lavandula angustifolia (lavender), Eucalyptus globulus (eucalyptus), Mentha piperita (peppermint), Rosmarinus officinalis (rosemary), Jasminum sambac (jasmine), Piper nigrum (black pepper) and so many other plants have neuroprotective effects.[267] Other studies mentioned the positive effects that citrus oils, including lemon and orange, can have on the brain.[268] As you can see, healthy brain function can be supported by a variety of nutritional and natural supplements.

MindWise™ was specially formulated with natural ingredients to support healthy brain function. This drink is made with a vegetarian oil made from cold-pressed sacha inchi seeds harvested from the Peruvian Amazon and other medium-chain triglyceride oils. Sacha inchi nuts have been used for centuries in Latin American countries to support brain health. Overall, MindWise™ has a high proportion of unsaturated fatty acids and omega-3 fatty acids. MindWise™ also contains a proprietary memory function blend made with bioidentical CoQ10, ALCAR, and GPC. Other ingredients in MindWise™ include turmeric, pomegranate fruit extract, rhododendron leaf extract, and vitamin D3. It also contains Peppermint, Lemon, Fennel, Lime, and Anise Essential Oils. It has no added preservatives. It's time to boost your brain and heart with MindWise™!

Note: None of the statements made about any of Young Living's products have been evaluated by the Food and Drug Administration. Young Living products are not intended to diagnose, treat, cure, or prevent any disease.

Most of the product information and text describing Young Living products is directly from Young Living Essential Oils, LC, and can be found online at youngliving.com

Brain Power™, KidScents®, GeneYus™, NingXia Nitro™, NingXia Zyng™, NingXia Red®, and MindWise™ are trademarks of Young Living Essential Oils, LC.

Month 6 Shopping List:

Product Name	Item Number	PV
NingXia Nitro™	3064	39.75
NingXia Zyng™	3071	26.75
MindWise™	21244	61.5
Total PV:		128
Bonus Essential Oil: Brain Power™		
For Your Kiddo: GeneYus™ Essential Oil		
Month 6 ER Points Earning Rate: 20%		
Rewards Points Earned this Month:		~25
Cumulative Reward Points:		~100

References:

[220] The world health report 2002 - reducing risks, promoting healthy life. World Health Organization WHO.

[221] World Health Organization WHO. Fact Sheets. Mental disorders. http://www.who.int/news-room/fact-sheets/detail/mental-disorders.

[222] GBD 2010: understanding disease, injury, and risk. Lancet. 2012 Dec 15;380(9859):2053-4. doi: 10.1016/S0140-6736(12)62133-3.

[223] Global Epidemiology of Dementia: Alzheimer's and Vascular Types. Biomed Res Int. 2014; 2014: 908915. doi: 10.1155/2014/908915.

[224] The Epidemiological Scale of Alzheimer's Disease. J Clin Med Res. 2015 Sep; 7(9): 657–666. doi: 10.14740/jocmr2106w.

[225] Lifetime prevalence of mental disorders in U.S. adolescents: results from the National Comorbidity Survey Replication--Adolescent Supplement (NCS-A). J Am Acad Child Adolesc Psychiatry. 2010 Oct;49(10):980-9. doi: 10.1016/j.jaac.2010.05.017.

[226] Gut Microbes and the Brain: Paradigm Shift in Neuroscience. J Neurosci. 2014 Nov 12; 34(46): 15490–15496. doi: 10.1523/JNEUROSCI.3299-14.2014.

[227] Psychobiotics and Their Involvement in Mental Health. J Mol Microbiol Biotechnol 2014;24:211-214. doi.org/10.1159/000366281.

[228] The aging mind: neuroplasticity in response to cognitive training. Dialogues Clin Neurosci. 2013 Mar; 15(1): 109–119. PMID: 23576894.

[229] Adult Neuroplasticity: More Than 40 Years of Research. Neural Plast. 2014; 2014: 541870. doi: 10.1155/2014/541870.

[230] Exercise Promotes Neuroplasticity in Both Healthy and Depressed Brains: An fMRI Pilot Study. Neural Plast. 2017; 2017: 8305287. doi: 10.1155/2017/8305287.

[231] Beneficial effects of physical exercise on neuroplasticity and cognition. Neurosci Biobehav Rev. 2013 Nov;37(9 Pt B):2243-57. doi: 10.1016/j.neubiorev.2013.04.005.

[232] Health Effects and Public Health Concerns of Energy Drink Consumption in the United States: A Mini-Review. Front Public Health. 2017; 5: 225. doi: 10.3389/fpubh.2017.00225.

[233] Energy drinks: Getting wings but at what health cost? Pak J Med Sci. 2014 Nov-Dec; 30(6): 1415–1419. doi: 10.12669/pjms.306.5396.

[234] Caffeine: Cognitive and Physical Performance Enhancer or Psychoactive Drug? Curr Neuropharmacol. 2015 Jan; 13(1): 71–88. doi: 10.2174/1570159 X13666141210215655.

[235] The Effect of Acute Consumption of Energy Drinks on Blood Pressure, Heart Rate and Blood Glucose in the Group of Young Adults. Int J Environ Res Public Health. 2018 Mar; 15(3): 544. doi: 10.3390/ijerph15030544.

[236] Cardiovascular complications from consumption of high energy drinks: recent evidence. J Hum Hypertens. 2015 Feb;29(2):71-6. doi: 10.1038/jhh.2014.47.

[237] The Effect of Acute Consumption of Energy Drinks on Blood Pressure, Heart Rate and Blood Glucose in the Group of Young Adults. Int J Environ Res Public Health. 2018 Mar; 15(3): 544. doi: 10.3390/ijerph15030544.

[238] Are energy drinks contributing to the obesity epidemic? Asia Pac J Clin Nutr. 2006;15(2):242-4. PMID: 16672210.

[239] Behavioral and physiologic adverse effects in adolescent and young adult emergency department patients reporting use of energy drinks and caffeine. Clin Toxicol (Phila). 2013 Aug;51(7):557-65. doi: 10.3109/15563650.2013.820311.

[240] Energy drinks: Getting wings but at what health cost? Pak J Med Sci. 2014 Nov-Dec; 30(6): 1415–1419. doi: 10.12669/pjms.306.5396.

[241] An analysis of energy-drink toxicity in the National Poison Data System. Clin Toxicol (Phila). 2013 Aug;51(7):566-74. doi: 10.3109/15563650.2013.820310.

[242] Energy drinks: health risks and toxicity. Med J Aust 2012; 196 (1): 46-49. || doi: 10.5694/mja11.10838.

[243] Update on Emergency Department Visits Involving Energy Drinks: A Continuing Public Health Concern. The CBHSQ Report. Rockville (MD):

Substance Abuse and Mental Health Services Administration (US); 2013. PMID: 27606410.

[244] An epidemic of energy? The case for stronger action on 'energy drinks'. Austr New Zea J Pub Health. doi.org/10.1111/1753-6405.12365.

[245] Health effects of energy drinks on children, adolescents, and young adults. Pediatrics. 2011 Mar;127(3):511-28. doi: 10.1542/peds.2009-3592.

[246] Neuroprotective and Anti-Aging Potentials of Essential Oils from Aromatic and Medicinal Plants. Front Aging Neurosci. 2017; 9: 168. doi: 10.3389/fnagi.2017.00168.

[247] Aromas of rosemary and lavender essential oils differentially affect cognition and mood in healthy adults. Int J Neurosci. 2003 Jan;113(1):15-38. PMID: 12690999.

[248] Modulation of cognitive performance and mood by aromas of peppermint and ylang-ylang. Int J Neurosci. 2008 Jan;118(1):59-77. PMID: 18041606 DOI: 10.1080/00207450601042094.

[249] Plasma 1,8-cineole correlates with cognitive performance following exposure to rosemary essential oil aroma. Ther Adv Psychopharmacol. 2012 Jun; 2(3): 103–113. doi: 10.1177/2045125312436573.

[250] Preliminary investigation of the effect of peppermint oil on an objective measure of daytime sleepiness. Int J Psychophysiol. 2005 Mar;55(3):291-8. PMID: 15708642 DOI: 10.1016/j.ijpsycho.2004.08.004.

[251] Effect of aromatherapy on patients with Alzheimer's disease PSYCHOGERIATRICS 2009; 9: 173–179. doi:10.1111/j.1479-8301.2009.00299.x.

[252] D-ribose--an additive with caffeine. Med Hypotheses. 2009 May;72(5):499-500. doi: 10.1016/j.mehy.2008.12.038.

[253] American Physiology Society. "Green Tea Extract Boosts Exercise Endurance 8-24%, Utilizing Fat As Energy Source." ScienceDaily. ScienceDaily, 31 January 2005. sciencedaily.com/releases/2005/01/050128221248.htm.

[254] Long-chain omega-3 fatty acids and the brain: a review of the independent and shared effects of EPA, DPA and DHA. Front Aging Neurosci. 2015; 7: 52. doi: 10.3389/fnagi.2015.00052.

[255] Neurological benefits of omega-3 fatty acids. Neuromolecular Med. 2008;10(4):219-35. doi: 10.1007/s12017-008-8036-z.

[256] Omega-3 dietary supplements and the risk of cardiovascular events: a systematic review. Clin Cardiol. 2009 Jul;32(7):365-72. doi: 10.1002/clc.20604.

[257] Omega-3 fatty acids and cardiovascular disease: effects on risk factors, molecular pathways, and clinical events. J Am Coll Cardiol. 2011 Nov 8;58(20):2047-67. doi: 10.1016/j.jacc.2011.06.063.

[258] Significance of long chain polyunsaturated fatty acids in human health. Clin Transl Med. 2017 Dec;6(1):25. doi: 10.1186/s40169-017-0153-6.

[259] Medium-Chain Fatty Acids Improve Cognitive Function in Intensively

Treated Type 1 Diabetic Patients and Support In Vitro Synaptic Transmission During Acute Hypoglycemia. Diabetes. 2009 May; 58(5): 1237–1244. doi: [10.2337/db08-1557].

[260] Dietary supplementation with medium-chain TAG has long-lasting cognition-enhancing effects in aged dogs. Br J Nutr. 2010 Jun;103(12):1746-54. doi: 10.1017/S0007114510000097.

[261] Effects of beta-hydroxybutyrate on cognition in memory-impaired adults. Send to Neurobiol Aging. 2004 Mar;25(3):311-4. DOI: 10.1016/S0197-4580(03)00087-3.

[262] Coenzyme Q10 administration increases brain mitochondrial concentrations and exerts neuroprotective effects. Proc Natl Acad Sci U S A. 1998 Jul 21; 95(15): 8892–8897. PMID: 9671775.

[263] ALCAR Exerts Neuroprotective and Pro-Neurogenic Effects by Inhibition of Glial Activation and Oxidative Stress via Activation of the Wnt/Beta-Catenin Signaling in Parkinsonian Rats. Mol Neurobiol. 2016 Sep;53(7):4286-301. doi: 10.1007/s12035-015-9361-5.

[264] Targeting Mitochondrial Dysfunction with L-Alpha Glycerylphosphorylcholine. PLoS One. 2016; 11(11): e0166682. doi: 10.1371/journal.pone.0166682.

[265] Vitamin D and cognitive function. Scand J Clin Lab Invest Suppl. 2012;243:79-82. doi: 10.3109/00365513.2012.681969.

[266] Vitamin D, cognitive dysfunction and dementia in older adults. CNS Drugs. 2011 Aug;25(8):629 39. doi: 10.2165/11593080-000000000-00000.

[267] Neuroprotective and Anti-Aging Potentials of Essential Oils from Aromatic and Medicinal Plants. Front Aging Neurosci. 2017; 9: 168. doi: [10.3389/fnagi.2017.00168].

[268] Biological Activities and Safety of Citrus spp. Essential Oils. Int J Mol Sci. 2018 Jul; 19(7): 1966. doi: [10.3390/ijms19071966].

♪CHAPTER 10

Month 7: Work It Out

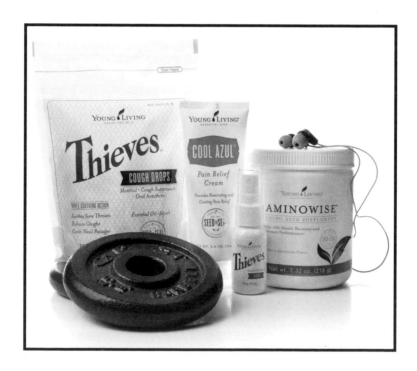

What if I could offer you a prescription that would lower your risk of getting cancer by at least 40-60% (depending on the type),[269] lower the progression to diabetes by 58%,[270] decrease the risk of dying from diabetes by up to 67%,[271] decrease the risk of getting dementia including Alzheimer's Disease by 45%,[272,273] decrease your risk of hip fractures by 55%,[274] and reduce moderate to severe mood disorders including depression by 47%?[275] In addition, you would also lower your risk of premature dying by 25%.[276] Would you accept such a prescription from Doctor Oli? Well, here it is: **Walk 30 minutes a day!** You can do it!

I know that you can do it. I had to do it myself, so I know with certainty that it can be done. When I moved to the United States from Switzerland, I quickly fell into the trap of consuming too much fast food, too often. After a short few years, I had gained a substantial amount of weight, and my blood values for sugar, fat, and inflammation markers went through the roof. First, I realized that I felt sluggish. Then came the breakouts on my face.

Finally, obesity set in. My overall health suffered. My heart started to widen, and its function progressively decreased. Like many people in the U.S., I started to use prescription medication to cover up for these shortcomings. It was not until I needed heart surgery that I woke up and realized this way of life had to stop.

With the help of my wife Ellen, I finally started to change my lifestyle. I started by walking 30 minutes a day, and then slowly increased that amount. After about eight months, I had lost almost 90 pounds, and I felt great! I no longer needed my prescription medications, and my blood tests showed normal values. Not to mention that I never had to undergo heart surgery as initially planned.

Literally, I walked the walk, and now I talk the talk. I know that it is not always easy and that there will be periods of no weight loss despite doing everything right. The name of the game is to not give up. Never, ever! Make your decision today, and go for it. I did it, and therefore you can as well. You will be glad you did it. Start by walking 30 minutes a day. Maybe the same thing that happened to me will happen to you. You might just start to enjoy your newfound health and fitness.

Today, I cannot imagine my life without my regular workouts. And my workouts are not anymore limited to the 30 minutes of brisk walking. You will read later in the chapter how I increased my athletic performance over time and what I do today to make these strenuous workout sessions more effective and enjoyable.

We all know about the importance of regular physical activity for children, teenagers, and adults including the elderly.[277] Men and women who reported increased levels of physical activity and fitness were found to have reductions of 20-35% in relative risk of death.[278,279] You probably heard some of the quotes attributed to Hippocrates (~450BC) such as "Walking is man's best medicine," "If there is any deficiency in food and exercise the body will fall sick," or "If we could give every individual the right amount of nourishment and exercise, not too little and not too much, we would have found the safest way to health."[280,281] The concept of using physical activity for wellness and health is not exactly a new one.

There is no doubt about the multiple benefits of cardiovascular and muscular fitness at any age, like prevention and reduction in cardiovascular diseases,[282,283] obesity,[284,285] type 2 diabetes,[286,287] metabolic syndromes,[288] cancers,[289,290,291] osteoporosis,[292] and depression.[293] In addition, other positive results include improving bodily health in terms of loss of memory,[294] cognitive function,[295] skeletal and muscular health,[296] mood swings,[297] hormone balance,[298] or lung function,[299] and more.[300]

Recent research also shows the impact fitness and physical exercise have on the microbiome, making them important tools to improve the diversity and richness of bacterial strains in the gut with all its resulting benefits on immune system, brain function, and overall wellbeing.[301,302,303]

On the other hand, we have plenty of scientific evidence that a lack of exercise is associated with chronic diseases and that physical inactivity has a large impact in shortening average life expectancy.[304] One interesting study looked at the impact of various factors on the prevention of cardiovascular disease. The authors analyzed several previous studies and compared the impacts of low fitness, obesity, smoking, high blood pressure, diabetes, and high cholesterol on overall cardiovascular health.

The results showed that not only did low fitness have the worst effects on cardiovascular health, it had a higher negative impact than obesity, smoking, diabetes, and high cholesterol combined.[305] Another study concluded that non-exercising 50-year-olds had twice the amount of chronic diseases than fit ones.[306]

We also know that approximately 11% of all healthcare expenditures in the United States are related directly to lack of exercise and inactivity.[307] A study looking at enrollees in a Minnesota health plan, age 40 or older, found that each additional "active" day per week resulted in a 4.7% decrease in health care cost. They concluded that five days of activity would represent about a 23.5% cost reduction compared with no days of physical activity.[308]

Lack of exercise, i.e. sedentary behavior, is a major cause of chronic diseases.[309] Sedentary behavior is defined as sitting or lying with low energy expenditure, not including sleep.[310] Time spent sitting, like at a desk, in front of the

TV, in a car, all increase risk of dying prematurely.[311] To meet the minimum effort to combat these dangers, all you need to do is limit sleeping and sitting to 23.5 hours a day, reserving only 30 minutes a day for exercise.

Many studies look at the type and amount of exercise necessary to decrease chronic diseases and risk of dying from several diseases. Options include aerobic versus anaerobic, strength exercises versus balance training, levels of intensity, and many others. These decisions go beyond the scope of this book.

To make it very simple, I recommend that you start with walking 30 minutes a day, every day. So even if you need to start with less time or a slower pace, just get going. You should now understand, without any doubt, that for optimal health, exercise is no longer optional. Check with your healthcare provider before starting any new exercises.

Of course, proper nutrition is important to support any physical activity. Over the last few decades, many resources have proposed differing ideas about the amount of consumption of each macronutrient (carbohydrates/sugars, lipids/fats, and amino acids/proteins). Hence the different diet plans such as low carb vs high carb, low fat vs high fat, and low protein vs high protein... or any combination of these. It is also noteworthy that one gram of sugar or protein yields about four calories, while one gram of fat yields about nine calories, which provides more energy per gram.

In general, people use too much sugar as an energy source and not enough protein and fat. This high sugar consumption can be blamed for many chronic diseases, and even an increased risk of dying. In fact, sugar-sweetened beverages are a marker of an unhealthy lifestyle, and people who drink them tend to consume more calories, exercise less, smoke more, and have a poor dietary pattern.[312]

When people exercise at a low to moderate intensity, like walking 30 minutes a day, they mostly use the oxidation of fatty acids as energy source. As energy requirements increase due to higher intensity of the physical activity, the body starts utilizing muscle glycogen (a special form of sugar stored mostly in the muscles), blood sugar, and intramuscular triglycerides to compensate.[313] Intensifying exercise will increase the use of muscle glycogen and also blood sugar until these sources are depleted.

Therefore, many professional athletes will consume higher amounts of sugars before, during, and after an athletic event. However, this use of sugars is done by highly trained and fit athletes and should not be compared with the use and abuse of sugars by the normal population. And even in the athletic world, there is a lot of discussion about what fuel sources might be the best option depending on the type of sport or athletic performance.

Recent scientific research found many advantages of low-carb/ketogenic diets (low sugar diets) in athletes reaching from better maximal oxygen uptake, maximal work load, to higher lactic threshold (the moment when muscles shut down due to lack of oxygen and too much lactic acid production).[314] An elevated fat oxidation rate and glycogen sparing effect may improve performance in ultra-endurance events.[315]

Both protein and fats can be converted to energy for our body. Proteins typically feed back into the glucose and glycogen producing pathways, while fats usually burndown to ketone bodies as the ultimate energy carrier, which is why a low carb, high fat/protein nutrition intake is called a ketogenic diet.

These metabolic effects support performance in later stages of high-intensity activity, during which aerobic (oxygen-dependent) metabolism becomes more important.

Ketogenic diets or lifestyles are also used very successfully these days for weight reduction.[316] Another advantage of this type of lifestyle is the decreased desire to eat, i.e. the appetite suppressant nature of such foods.[317] Together with increased exercise, a ketogenic food plan might have a significant effect on achieving optimal body weight, reducing fat mass, improving lean muscle mass, improving central nervous and peripheral nervous function, as well as improving overall wellness. Ketogenic diets also have the potential to help treat a variety of diseases, including cancer.[318]

If your overall sugar/carbohydrate intake is reduced, what kind of fuel source should you use instead? Well, the two options left are proteins and fats. Both can be found in various types of foods but can also be supplemented in times of need. A good fat-based supplement would likely come in the form of medium-chained triglycerides (found in MindWise™ for example), as these types of fats increase mitochondrial biogenesis (the creation of more energy factories within the cells) and are also relatively easily metabolized by the body and will provide a good energy source.[319]

However, muscle mass is mostly determined by the synthesis and breakdown of protein in the muscle.[320] This process can be significantly changed by adding exercise to the mix. Proteins are by definition poly-peptides (clusters of peptides). Peptides are chains made of various amino acids. We can classify the 21 human amino acids into three groups: essential, non-essential, and conditional amino acids.[321]

Essential amino acids have to be consumed since they cannot be produced by the body, hence the name essential. The nine essential amino acids are histidine, isoleucine, leucine, lysine, methionine, phenylalanine, threonine, tryptophan, and valine.

Non-essential amino acids are produced in our bodies but are still essential for the body to function. The four non-essential amino acids are alanine, asparagine, aspartic acid, and glutamic acid.

Conditional amino acids are usually not essential, except in times of illness and stress. The eight conditional amino acids are arginine, cysteine, glutamine, tyrosine, glycine, ornithine, proline, and serine.

Amino acids can come from animal sources (mostly complete amino acid profiles) or from plant-based compounds (mostly incomplete amino acid profiles). To summarize, amino acids are the building blocks of proteins and the proteins are the building blocks of life.

It is well-known that during the normal process of aging, humans start losing muscle mass. The medical term used to describe the slow but progressive reduction of muscle mass is sarcopenia. The impact of lack of nutritional elements on morbidity (getting sick) and mortality (dying from the disease) is unquestionable.

Malnutrition increases the risk for frailty and nutritional deficits can influence immune status, response to medical treatments and recovery from acute illnesses, including surgery.[322] In 2000, 18.5 billion U.S. dollars in health care expenditures were directly attributable to sarcopenia.[323] A lack of protein in the elderly population is also associated with lower family function scores.[324] Adequate protein intake is also very important for infants and children to assure their normal development.

Protein supplementation is very popular amongst those who exercise and can make up to 50% or more of their supplementation products.[325] Protein supplementation alone has not clearly proven to improve overall muscle mass.

However, when combined with fitness it will usually do the trick,[326,327] and the need for good protein increases when exercising.[328,329,330] Also, recent evidence indicates that ingesting protein and/or amino acids prior to, during, and/or following exercise can enhance recovery, immune function, and growth and maintenance of lean body mass.[331]

Proper amounts of amino acids are required for the optimal synthesis and concentration of a variety of immune related proteins and a good functioning immune system. Together with a healthy microbiome, also supported by regular exercise,[332] the immune system just might get the boost it needs.[333] With all of this in mind, I recommend adding some of Young Living's protein products (like AminoWise™ or Pure Protein™ Complete) to this month's suggested Essential Rewards order to support your healthy exercise performance.

AminoWise™

Young Living created the protein/mineral blend AminoWise™ by combining three support mechanisms for your healthy physical activity: the Muscle Performance blend aids muscle building and repair, the Recovery blend helps reduce muscle fatigue, and the Hydration Mineral blend replenishes important minerals lost during exercise. A synergistic complex of amino acids and antioxidants helps with fatigue and enhances muscle recovery during and after exercise, while an antioxidant and mineral complex was added to help reduce lactic acid levels induced by exercise. AminoWise™ also supports the production of nitric oxide, which can improve vascular blood flow.

Its Muscle Performance blend contains branched chain amino acids (BCAA's) leucine, iso-leucine, and valine, which all have shown to aid in preventing muscle catabolism from exercise. For humans, the three muscle-supporting BCAA's are part of the nine essential amino acids. The formula also contains other muscle-supporting amino acids such as L-citrulline, L-glutamine, B-alanine, L-arginine, and L-taurine.

The Recovery blend was formulated using Ningxia wolfberry and lime fruit powders, Lemon and Lime Essential Oils, polyphenol extract, as well as zinc and vitamin E.

The Hydration Mineral blend contains sodium citrate, potassium citrate, calcium citrate, and magnesium citrate.

Together with water, used to dissolve the blend into a tasty drink, these minerals support healthy hydration by replenishing important minerals lost during exercise when taken during or after your workout. AminoWise™ does not contain any preservatives, synthetic colors, or artificial flavors, nor does it have added sugars or artificial sweeteners. AminoWise™ is a very special and unique product in the field of workout supplementation.

In addition to the research on protein supplementation, there are numerous scientific studies researching the use of essential oils during exercise and athletic performance. A clear star here seems to be peppermint essential oil. Since peppermint essential oil has been registered as dietary supplement by Young Living, function-structure claims citing the appropriate references in scientific literature are permitted (at least in the U.S.). One study described the effectiveness of peppermint essential oil on exercise performance, gas analysis, spirometry parameters, blood pressure, as well as respiratory rate.[334]

Another study measured several strength and performance parameters as well as respiratory function after ingestion of peppermint essential oil. The authors showed a significant increase in the grip force (36.1%), standing vertical jump (7.0%), and standing long jump (6.4%) in those using the essential oil.[335] Lung function measurements revealed significant positive changes for those ingesting peppermint essential oil including increase in the forced vital capacity in the first second (FVC1) (35.1%), peak inspiratory flow rate (PIF) (66.4%), and peak expiratory flow rate (PEF) (65.1%), all of these being important parameters of respiratory function.

In addition, the results also showed a positive effect on visual and audio reaction times as well as on the "time to exhaustion" parameter during physical exercise. It has also been shown that the positive effects of peppermint odor in regard to vigilance of athletes resulted in better overall athletic performance.[336] Other authors exhibited that peppermint essential oil could powerfully relieve exercise-induced fatigue.[337] Yet another study found that the topical application of orange and/or spearmint essential oils also improved exercise performance and respiratory function parameters.[338]

Now let's have a look to see what else could be added to your Essential Rewards order in a month dedicated to physical exercise and cardiovascular fitness...while at the same time learning a few tricks from Doctor Oli support your natural, doping-free performance enhancement.

Cool Azul™ Pain Relief Cream

Many pain relief creams are made with harsh chemicals and synthetic ingredients. Young Living formulated the Cool Azul™ Pain Relief Cream as a healthy alternative to these commercial products. It provides cooling relief from minor muscle and joint aches, arthritis, strains, bruises, and sprains. It is also a perfect product to use before and after workout sessions. Cool Azul™ Pain Relief Cream is made with the Cool Azul™ Essential Oil blend (Wintergreen, Peppermint, Sage, Copaiba, Oregano, Melaleuca, Lavender, Blue Cypress, Elemi, Vetiver, Caraway, Dorado Azul™, and Chamomile) combined with additional Wintergreen and

Peppermint Essential Oils. Other natural ingredients in this product are green tea leaf extract, rosehip seed oil, mango butter, and aloe leaf juice.

Use the cream prior to exercise, and you will quickly feel the heating effect it has on your muscles. After a workout, the natural methyl salicylate found in wintergreen helps alleviate pain deep in the muscles and joints, while the natural menthol found in peppermint provides a cooling effect. By combining methyl salicylate with natural menthol, this pain relief cream offers a unique topical analgesic infused with Young Living's 100% pure, therapeutic grade essential oils and other plant-based ingredients for effective temporary pain relief.

Thieves® Spray

Before and after a workout session, you should sanitize your exercise equipment and the surrounding area. Thieves® Spray is small and handy and uses only naturally derived, plant-based ingredients combined with the powerful spicy-citrus scent of Thieves® Essential Oil blend. It enables a quick cleaning of your workout space. Simply spray the surfaces a couple times, let it dry, or wipe the area with a clean towel or a Thieves® or Seedlings™ wipe. Et voilà, you are ready to go! If you do this after working out as well, anyone using the exercise machine next will appreciate having a clean piece of equipment.

Thieves® Cough Drops

Experience the power of Thieves® and menthol in a cough drop! The triple-action formula of Thieves® Cough Drops offers comfort by relieving coughs, soothing sore throats, and cooling nasal passages. Minty, spicy, and sweet without processed sugar, dyes, artificial flavors, or preservatives, these cough drops are made with naturally derived ingredients, including menthol (8 mg) and

Cinnamon Bark, Clove, Eucalyptus, Lemon, Peppermint, and Rosemary Essential Oils. Other ingredients are stevia leaf extract, pectin, and water. These tasty cough drops are easy to take anywhere you may need relief. Keep some in your purse, laptop bag, gym bag, or next to your bed at night so they're always on hand to soothe. Keep reading to find out how I incorporate these cough drops into my workout preparations!

Doctor Oli's Workout Regimen

How do I, Doctor Oli, prepare for most of my exercise sessions? First, I want to say that I often use an almost extreme preparation for my workout. This reflects the joy I now experience after having lost so much weight, resulting in significantly better health. You can simply walk 30 minutes a day. Or, start increasing your athletic performance by adding one or more of the following techniques.

I start by turning on one or two diffusers with Peppermint Essential Oil, Northern Lights Black Spruce Essential Oil, and Idaho Blue Spruce Essential Oil at least 20 minutes prior to my session. Eucalyptus, RC™, or any other essential oil or blend supporting healthy breathing would also be a good choice. I also often apply Breathe Again™ Roll-On topically to my chest. Then, I mix coconut milk, which is rich in the energy source medium-chained triglycerides, with Young Living's Pure Protein™ Complete powder, to fuel up my ATP and energy levels.

While enjoying my protein drink, I go through my oil application routine. There are a few steps to it, but the results are great! First, I topically apply the following essential oils on my muscles to preheat for my upcoming workout: Wintergreen, Copaiba, Peppermint, and any of the blends PanAway™, Aroma Siez™, Cool Azul™, or Deep Relief™. Also, I often topically apply Golden Rod, Idaho Blue Spruce, Mister™, Nutmeg, and Grapefruit Essential

Oils to support healthy male hormone balance and healthy metabolism.

Next, I spray floral water (the water from the essential oil distillation process which contains some plant material) on top of the oils. If you do not have floral water, you could just use regular water. Remember, application of water typically increases the effect of essential oils, so never use water to soothe a spot where an essential oil might be giving you a warming sensation like lips, eyes, or sensitive skin areas.

After the floral water spray, I apply either Cool Azul™ Gel or Cool Azul™ Pain Cream (or both!) to seal off the previously applied essential oils in order to prevent evaporation of the oils into the air.

Before prepping my muscles, I pop a Thieves® Cough Drop into my mouth in order feel the freshness and air flow going through my nose and mouth into my lungs. This effect happens because menthol directly stimulates cold receptors modulating the cool sensation, resulting in a subjective feeling of a clear and wide nose and airway.[339] Menthol also can improve athletic performance mainly through its core temperature lowering properties.[340] Just make sure that the cough drop completely dissolves before you start your workout session to avoid choking!

While the Thieves® Cough Drop dissolves, and the essential oils on my muscles take effect, I prepare my sports drink. I frequently change the recipe for this drink, but I almost always use at least one NingXia Nitro®, a little NingXia Red® as an antioxidant, a scoop of AminoWise™, and one drop of Peppermint Essential Oil, often accompanied by one drop of Black Pepper Essential Oil.

Sometimes I will even add a few drops of one of the citrus essential oils into the drink. It tastes great and supports healthy detoxing while I sweat out some of the toxins. This occurs in the later stages of a workout session, when my body temperature is higher and the essential oils and Cool Azul™ cream have absorbed into my body.

Again, before your workout begins, be sure the Thieves® Cough Drop is fully dissolved to avoid choking or inhaling it into the windpipe. During my workout, which is usually a couple hours of walking/running, I sip on my drink and sometimes add an additional layer of some of the essential oils to my strained muscles after about 30 minutes of exercise. The steady inhalation of the aromatically diffused essential oils feels great when I start breathing more heavily.

After I'm done working out, I'll hop in the shower and use any of Young Living's shampoos and body washes (they are, as you now know, formulated without toxins). Then, I topically apply Copaiba Essential Oil and Cool Azul™ Gel or Pain Relief Cream to support healthy recovery of my muscles. Sometimes I will make and enjoy another small portion of coconut milk with Pure Protein™ Complete Chocolate powder since studies have shown that the consumption of chocolate milk after exercise improves recovery.[341,342,343]

So, there you have it! Use these tricks and your next exercise session will be more enjoyable. Ditch your sedentary behaviors, switch to a more active lifestyle, and refresh your body and overall wellness by enjoying the benefits gained from increased physical activity. Oh, and I forgot to mention that over time, you will look significantly healthier, stronger, and more attractive. What's not to love about that?

Note: None of the statements made about any of Young Living's products have been evaluated by the Food and Drug Administration. Young Living products are not intended to diagnose, treat, cure, or prevent any disease.

Most of the product information and text describing Young Living products is directly from Young Living Essential Oils, LC, and can be found online at youngliving.com

Deep Relief™, KidScents®, MightyVites™, MindWise™, AminoWise™, Pure Protein™, Cool Azul™, Dorado Azul™, Thieves®, RC™, PanAway™, Aroma Siez™, Cool Azul™, Mister™, NingXia Nitro®, and NingXia Red® are trademarks of Young Living Essential Oils, LC.

Month 7 Shopping List:

Product Name	Item Number	PV
AminoWise™	20083	33.75
Thieves® Essential Oil Infused Cough Drops	5760	20.5
Cool Azul™ Pain Relief Cream	5759	44
Thieves® Spray	3265	9.25
	Total PV:	107.5
Bonus Essential Oil: Deep Relief™ Roll-On		
For Your Kiddo: MightyVites™ Chewable Tablets		
Month 7 ER Points Earning Rate: 20%		
Rewards Points Earned this Month:		~21
Cumulative Reward Points:		~121

References:

[269] Adherence to Diet and Physical Activity Cancer Prevention Guidelines and Cancer Outcomes: A Systematic Review. Cancer Epidemiol Biomarkers Prev. 2016 Jul; 25(7): 1018–1028. doi: 10.1158/1055-9965.EPI-16-0121.

[270] Exercise and Type 2 Diabetes. Diabetes Care. 2010 Dec; 33(12): e147–e167. doi: 10.2337/dc10-9990.

[271] Exercise capacity and all-cause mortality in African American and Caucasian men with type 2 diabetes. Diabetes Care. 2009 Apr;32(4):623-8. doi: 10.2337/dc08-1876.

[272] Alzheimer's disease: Can exercise prevent memory loss? Mayo Clinic.

[273] Physical activity and risk of neurodegenerative disease: a systematic review of prospective evidence. Psychol Med. 2009 Jan;39(1):3-11. doi: 10.1017/S0033291708003681.

[274] Walking and Leisure-Time Activity and Risk of Hip Fracture in Postmenopausal Women. JAMA. 2002;288(18):2300-2306. doi:10.1001/jama.288.18.2300.

[275] Exercise treatment for depression: efficacy and dose response. Am J Prev Med. 2005 Jan;28(1):1-8. DOI: 10.1016/j.amepre.2004.09.003.

[276] World Health Organization WHO. Physical activity. http://www.who.int/news-room/fact-sheets/detail/physical-activity.

[277] Physical fitness in childhood and adolescence: a powerful marker of health. Int J Obes (Lond). 2008 Jan;32(1):1-11. DOI: 10.1038/sj.ijo.0803774.

[278] Population attributable risk: implications of physical activity dose. Med Sci Sports Exerc. 2001 Jun;33(6 Suppl):S635-9; discussion 640-1. PMID: 11427788.

[279] Major public health benefits of physical activity. Arthritis Rheum. 2003 Feb 15;49(1):122-8. DOI: 10.1002/art.10907.

[280] Brainy Quotes. Hippocrates Quotes.

281 The Hippocratic concept of positive health in the 5th century BC and in the new millennium. World Rev Nutr Diet. 2001;89:1-4. PMID: 11530728.

[282] Cardiovascular benefits of exercise. Int J Gen Med. 2012; 5: 541–545. doi: 10.2147/IJGM.S30113.

[283] Exercise and heart disease in women: why, how, and how much? Cardiol Rev. 1999 Sep-Oct;7(5):301-8. PMID: 11208241.

[284] Physical activity in obesity and metabolic syndrome. Ann N Y Acad Sci. 2013 Apr; 1281(1): 141–159. doi: 10.1111/j.1749-6632.2012.06785.x.

[285] Physical activity and gain in abdominal adiposity and body weight: prospective cohort study in 288,498 men and women. Am J Clin Nutr. 2011 Apr;93(4):826-35. doi: 10.3945/ajcn.110.006593.

[286] Exercise in obesity, metabolic syndrome, and diabetes. Prog Cardiovasc Dis. 2011 May-Jun;53(6):412-8. doi: 10.1016/j.pcad.2011.03.013.

[287] Resistance training for obese, type 2 diabetic adults: a review of the evidence. Obes Rev. 2010 Oct;11(10):740-9. doi: 10.1111/j.1467-789X.2009.00692.x.

[288] Exercise in the Metabolic Syndrome. Oxid Med Cell Longev. 2012; 2012: 349710. doi: 10.1155/2012/349710.

[289] Exercise and cancer: from "healthy" to "therapeutic"? Cancer Immunol Immunother. 2017; 66(5): 667–671. doi: 10.1007/s00262-017-1985-z.

[290] Voluntary Running Suppresses Tumor Growth through Epinephrine- and IL-6-Dependent NK Cell Mobilization and Redistribution. Cell Metab. 2016 Mar 8;23(3):554-62. doi: 10.1016/j.cmet.2016.01.011.

[291] Molecular Mechanisms Linking Exercise to Cancer Prevention

and Treatment. Cell Metab. 2018 Jan 9;27(1):10-21. doi: 10.1016/j. cmet.2017.09.015.

[292] Osteoporosis and exercise. Postgrad Med J. 2003 Jun; 79(932): 320–323. doi: 10.1136/pmj.79.932.320.

[293] Exercise as a treatment for depression: A meta-analysis adjusting for publication bias. J Psychiatr Res. 2016 Jun;77:42-51. doi: 10.1016/j. jpsychires.2016.02.023.

[294] The Effects of Exercise on Memory Function Among Young to Middle-Aged Adults: Systematic Review and Recommendations for Future Research. Am J Health Promot. 2018 Mar;32(3):691-704. doi: 10.1177/0890117117737409.

[295] The Influence of Exercise on Cognitive Abilities. Compr Physiol. 2013 Jan; 3(1): 403–428. doi: 10.1002/cphy.c110063.

[296] Exercise and physical health: musculoskeletal health and functional capabilities. Res Q Exerc Sport. 1995 Dec;66(4):276-85. DOI: 10.1080/02701367.1995.10607912.

[297] Physical Exercise for Treatment of Mood Disorders: A Critical Review. Curr Behav Neurosci Rep. 2016 Dec; 3(4): 350–359. doi: 10.1007/s40473-016-0089-y.

[298] Hormonal alterations due to exercise. Sports Med. 1986 Sep-Oct;3(5):331-45. PMID: 3529282.

[299] Effects of Aerobic Exercise on Lung Function in Overweight and Obese Students. Tanaffos. 2011; 10(3): 24–31. PMID: 25191372.

[300] Center for Disease Control and Prevention CDC. The Benefits of Physical Activity. https://www.cdc.gov/physicalactivity/basics/pa-health/index.htm.

[301] Exercise Modifies the Gut Microbiota with Positive Health Effects. Oxid Med Cell Longev. 2017; 2017: 3831972. doi: 10.1155/2017/3831972.

[302] Physical exercise, gut, gut microbiota, and atherosclerotic cardiovascular diseases. Lipids Health Dis. 2018; 17: 17. PMID: 29357881.

[303] Exercise Alters Gut Microbiota Composition and Function in Lean and Obese Humans. Med Sci Sports Exerc. 2018 Apr;50(4):747-757. doi: 10.1249/MSS.0000000000001495.

[304] Lifetime sedentary living accelerates some aspects of secondary aging. J Appl Physiol (1985). 2011 Nov;111(5):1497-504. doi: 10.1152/japplphysiol.00420.2011.

[305] Physical activity and the prevention of cardiovascular disease: from evolution to epidemiology. Prog Cardiovasc Dis. 2011 May-Jun;53(6):387-96. doi: 10.1016/j.pcad.2011.02.006.

[306] Midlife Fitness and the Development of Chronic Conditions in Later Life. Arch Intern Med. 2012 Sep 24; 172(17): 1333–1340. doi: 10.1001/archinternmed.2012.3400.

[307] Inadequate Physical Activity and Health Care Expenditures in the United States. Prog Cardiovasc Dis. 2015 Jan-Feb; 57(4): 315–323. doi: 10.1016/j. pcad.2014.08.002.

[308] Relationship between modifiable health risks and short-term health care charges. JAMA. 1999 Dec 15;282(23):2235-9. PMID: 10605975.

[309] Lack of exercise is a major cause of chronic diseases. Compr Physiol. 2012 Apr; 2(2): 1143–1211. doi: 10.1002/cphy.c110025.

[310] 24 Hours of Sleep, Sedentary Behavior, and Physical Activity with Nine Wearable Devices. Med Sci Sports Exerc. 2016 Mar; 48(3): 457–465. doi: 10.1249/MSS.0000000000000778.

[311] Too much sitting: the population health science of sedentary behavior. Exerc Sport Sci Rev. 2010 Jul;38(3):105-13. doi: 10.1097/JES.0b013e3181e373a2.

[312] Controversies about sugars: results from systematic reviews and meta-analyses on obesity, cardiometabolic disease and diabetes. Eur J Nutr. 2016 Nov;55(Suppl 2):25-43. doi: 10.1007/s00394-016-1345-3.

[313] Substrate utilization during exercise in active people. Am J Clin Nutr. 1995 Apr;61(4 Suppl):968S-979S. doi: 10.1093/ajcn/61.4.968S.

[314] The Effects of a Ketogenic Diet on Exercise Metabolism and Physical Performance in Off-Road Cyclists. Nutrients. 2014 Jul; 6(7): 2493–2508. doi: 10.3390/nu6072493.

[315] Low-Carbohydrate-High-Fat Diet: Can it Help Exercise Performance? J Hum Kinet. 2017 Mar 12;56:81-92. doi: 10.1515/hukin-2017-0025.

[316] Very-low-carbohydrate ketogenic diet v. low-fat diet for long-term weight loss: a meta-analysis of randomised controlled trials. Br J Nutr. 2013 Oct;110(7):1178-87. doi: 10.1017/S0007114513000548.

[317] Do ketogenic diets really suppress appetite? A systematic review and meta-analysis. Obes Rev. 2015 Jan;16(1):64-76. doi: 10.1111/obr.12230.

[318] Beyond weight loss: a review of the therapeutic uses of very-low-carbohydrate (ketogenic) diets. Eur J Clin Nutr. 2013 Aug; 67(8): 789–796. doi: 10.1038/ejcn.2013.116.

[319] Medium Chain Triglycerides enhances exercise endurance through the increased mitochondrial biogenesis and metabolism. PLoS One. 2018; 13(2): e0191182. doi: 10.1371/journal.pone.0191182.

[320] Role of dietary protein in the sarcopenia of aging. Am J Clin Nutr. 2008 May;87(5):1562S-1566S. DOI: 10.1093/ajcn/87.5.1562S.

[321] U.S. National Library of Medicine. Amino acids. https://medlineplus.gov/ency/article/002222.htm.

[322] Protein and amino acid supplementation in older humans. Amino Acids. 2013 Jun;44(6):1493-509. doi: 10.1007/s00726-013-1480-6.

[323] Dietary implications on mechanisms of sarcopenia: roles of protein, amino acids and antioxidants. J Nutr Biochem. 2010 Jan;21(1):1-13. doi: 10.1016/j.jnutbio.2009.06.014.

[324] Association between sarcopenia with lifestyle and family function among community-dwelling Chinese aged 60 years and older. BMC Geriatr. 2017 Aug 18;17(1):187. doi: 10.1186/s12877-017-0587-0.

[325] Prevalence of Dietary Supplements Use among Gymnasium Users.

Journal of Nutrition and Metabolism Volume 2017, Article ID 9219361, https://doi.org/10.1155/2017/9219361.

[326] The effects of protein supplements on muscle mass, strength, and aerobic and anaerobic power in healthy adults: a systematic review. Sports Med. 2015 Jan;45(1):111-31. doi: 10.1007/s40279-014-0242-2.

[327] A systematic review, meta-analysis and meta-regression of the effect of protein supplementation on resistance training-induced gains in muscle mass and strength in healthy adults. Br J Sports Med. 2018 Mar;52(6):376-384. doi: 10.1136/bjsports-2017-097608.

[328] Protein Requirements Are Elevated in Endurance Athletes after Exercise as Determined by the Indicator Amino Acid Oxidation Method. PLoS One. 2016; 11(6): e0157406. doi: 10.1371/journal.pone.0157406.

[329] Increased Protein Requirements in Female Athletes after Variable-Intensity Exercise. Med Sci Sports Exerc. 2017 Nov;49(11):2297-2304. doi: 10.1249/MSS.0000000000001366.

[330] Do athletes need more dietary protein and amino acids? Int J Sport Nutr. 1995 Jun;5 Suppl:S39-61. PMID: 7550257.

[331] Protein for exercise and recovery. Phys Sportsmed. 2009 Jun;37(2):13-21. doi: 10.3810/psm.2009.06.1705.

[332] Exercise and associated dietary extremes impact on gut microbial diversity. Gut. 2014 Dec;63(12):1913-20. doi: 10.1136/gutjnl-2013-306541.

[333] Exercise and gut immune function: evidence of alterations in colon immune cell homeostasis and microbiome characteristics with exercise training. Immunol Cell Biol. 2016 Feb;94(2):158-63. doi: 10.1038/icb.2015.108.

[334] The effects of peppermint on exercise performance. J Int Soc Sports Nutr. 2013; 10: 15. doi: 10.1186/1550-2783-10-15.

[335] Instant effects of peppermint essential oil on the physiological parameters and exercise performance. Avicenna J Phytomed. 2014 Jan;4(1):72-8. PMID: 25050303.

[336] The Effects of Odors on Objective and Subjective Measures of Athletic Performance. International Sports Journal; Winter2002, Vol. 6 Issue 1, p14.

[337] Does the Fragrance of Essential Oils Alleviate the Fatigue Induced by Exercise? Evid Based Complement Alternat Med. 2017; 2017: 5027372. doi: 10.1155/2017/5027372.

[338] The effect of inhalation of Citrus sinensis flowers and Mentha spicata leave essential oils on lung function and exercise performance: a quasi-experimental uncontrolled before-and-after study. J Int Soc Sports Nutr. 2016; 13: 36. doi: 10.1186/s12970-016-0146-7.

[339] Impact of menthol inhalation on nasal mucosal temperature and nasal patency. Am J Rhinol. 2008 Jul-Aug;22(4):402-5. doi: 10.2500/ajr.2008.22.3194.

[340] Menthol: A Fresh Ergogenic Aid for Athletic Performance. Sports Med. 2017 Jun;47(6):1035-1042. doi: 10.1007/s40279-016-0652-4.

[341] Chocolate milk as a post-exercise recovery aid. Int J Sport Nutr Exerc Metab. 2006 Feb;16(1):78-91. PMID: 16676705.

[342] Chocolate milk: a post-exercise recovery beverage for endurance sports. Med Sport Sci. 2012;59:127-34. doi: 10.1159/000341954.

[343] Improved endurance capacity following chocolate milk consumption compared with 2 commercially available sport drinks. Appl Physiol Nutr Metab. 2009 Feb;34(1):78-82. doi: 10.1139/H08-137.

CHAPTER 11

Month 8: Spoil Yourself

For the Gentlemen

For the Ladies

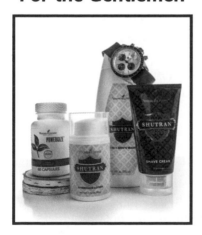
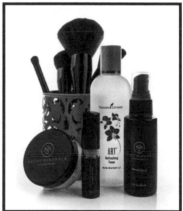

It's time to spoil yourself! While healthy lifestyle choices will lift your spirits and support a healthy hormone balance, I have a few additional suggestions on how both men and women can use Young Living's healthy products to further boost self-confidence and make their inner and outer beauty shine even more. For the ladies, non-toxic beauty products, like makeup, that are formulated without toxins, are a nice way to reward yourself. For the gentlemen, I looked for products that support masculinity, athletic performance, and healthy male hormone balance. And as a bonus, I've included some scientific evidence on how to support healthy hair growth for women and men.

For the Ladies

Admittedly, I am not an expert on the application of cosmetics or beauty tips. Whenever I don't know too much about something, I research it! So, in March of 2018, I attended a Young Living Beauty School event in Dallas to get some hands-on education about this topic. I highly recommend that both women and men attend a Beauty School event, because you learn so much about the uses and applications of Young Living's cosmetics and skin care products. My wife, daughter, and daughter-in-law have also taught me so much, so I'd like to thank them for their input for this chapter.

Now that you've changed your habits and created a mostly toxin-free household, it's time to finish this task by tossing out your highly noxious makeups and beauty products. Most women use makeup to appear younger, but while doing so, the harsh chemicals in those products not only significantly increase the toxic burden on the body and the environment, but they also accelerate the skin's aging process. This results in needing to use more of these bad beauty products to cover the damage from the ones you used before, and the vicious cycle continues.

The group Environmental Defense tested 49 different makeup items, including foundations, concealers, powders, blushes, mascaras, eye liners, eye shadows, lipsticks, and lip glosses. Their testing revealed serious heavy metal contamination in virtually all the products: 100% contained nickel, 96% contained lead, 90% contained beryllium, 61% contained thallium, 51% contained cadmium, and 20% contained arsenic.[344] And women apply these products not just once in their lifetime, but almost every day for decades!

But cosmetics do not just contain heavy metals, they also include synthetic colors (derived from coal tar), phthalates, parabens, sodium lauryl sulfate (SLS), sodium laureth sulfate (SLES), formaldehyde and formaldehyde-releasing preservatives, triclosan, diethanolamine (DEA) and triethanolamine, PEG compounds, propylene glycol (used also in antifreeze and to create artificial smoke),[345] talc, petroleum/paraffin/mineral oil, fragrances or flavor, toluene and butylated hydroxytoluene (BHT), butylated hydroxyanisole (BHA), siloxanes, imidazolidinyl urea, and the list goes on and on.

The United States Federal Food, Drug, and Cosmetic Act (FFDCA, FDCA, or FD&C) is a set of laws passed by Congress in 1938 to allow the Food and Drug Administration (FDA) to oversee the safety of food, drugs, and cosmetics. When it comes to cosmetics, manufacturers are not required to make a full disclosure of ingredients on the label. The FDA only requires cosmetics to have an "ingredient declaration," a list of all the product's ingredients.

The FDA requires this labeling under the Fair Packaging and Labeling Act (FPLA). But according to the FPLA, regulations for this list of ingredients must not be used to force a company to disclose "trade secrets." For example, fragrance and flavor ingredients do not need to be listed individually on cosmetic labels, because they are the ingredients most likely to be "trade secrets." Instead, those may be listed simply as "fragrance" or "flavor."[346] The term "fragrance" refers to a non-disclosed mixture that may be composed of any of over 3,000 chemicals, including allergens and reproductive toxins.

In other words, if you do not see some toxic or potentially toxic ingredients on a label of a cosmetic, that does not mean that they are not in the product. The FDA does not have the legal authority to proactively approve cosmetic products and ingredients (other than color additives) before they go on the market.[347] They only react to complaints after consumers report harmful side effects.

Therefore, it is up to the consumer to a) realize that they were harmed by something that is potentially not disclosed on the labels of their beauty products and is therefore unknown to them, b) make the connection between short-term or long-term adverse effect of a cosmetic on their body, and c) to figure out how to correctly report something about an ingredient they didn't even know existed in their products. Doesn't that make you want to use cosmetics that are made without harsh chemicals and fully disclose their ingredients on the label?

To give you healthier alternatives to the cosmetics and products currently available, Young Living has several options for skin care based on your personal needs. The first skin care line they created was ART® (Age Refining Technology), an entire system of beauty products. Later on, Young Living formulated other skin care options, like the Orange Blossom line that I mentioned in Month 4. And Young Living has a complete makeup line called Savvy Minerals by Young Living™, which is basically made from ground-up stones, vegetables, plants, and tree bark. They are completely safe to use and are not tested on animals. Young Living's products are all cruelty-free.

Savvy Minerals by Young Living™ Makeup: Foundation, Misting Spray, and Lipstick

Get confidence without compromise with Young Living's pure, natural, high-quality, mineral-based makeup line. Young Living believes in empowering women to stand out in their own unique, natural beauty, with help from products they can feel good about using. Unlike most mineral powders, Savvy Minerals cosmetics are made from plants and stones and are therefore free from cheap fillers and additives. These are natural makeup products that deliver rich colors with a smooth, luxurious application.

Whether you use the Savvy Minerals Foundation as an individual product for a more natural approach, or as the base of an elaborate look, it's got you covered. Savvy Minerals Foundation is made with high-quality, mineral-based ingredients. Its buildable formula can be used for sheer to full coverage and blends flawlessly for a natural-looking foundation that still diminishes the appearance of imperfections and blemishes.

It is also an all-day foundation, so you don't need to worry about it as you transition between your home, work, and social life. Plus, it was specially crafted without fillers, synthetics, or parabens, making it a great foundation for sensitive skin. With its long-lasting formula, gentle ingredients, and gorgeous finish, Savvy Minerals Foundation is the only coverage you need stashed in your makeup bag. Savvy Minerals Foundations are organized by undertones and shades.

The warm colors complement yellow, peach, or golden undertones, while the cool colors are best for pink or red undertones. The dark colors have neutral undertones. Each tone (Warm, Cool, and Dark), comes in various shades, with No. 1 as the lightest. As the number goes up, the shade gets darker. Once you know your undertone and preferred shade, you're ready to start building your perfect look. Overall, the foundation powder minimizes pore appearance, brightens complexion, absorbs excess oils, enhances natural beauty, is ideal for sensitive skin, is vegan-friendly, and is cruelty-free. It was formulated with mica, boron nitride, lauroyl lysine (an amino acid made from natural coconut oil), aspen bark extract, kaolin clay, and silica.

Take control of your makeup application with the Savvy Minerals by Young Living™ Misting Spray. Made with pure essential oils and plant-based ingredients, this aromatic Misting Spray gives you more control with your mineral powder makeup application, so you'll look and smell amazing. It helps with mineral powder application. Simply spray an applicator brush a few times before applying powder for even, thorough, and silky coverage. This product has a light, uplifting fragrance with hints of Lavender, Cedarwood, and Rose Essential Oils. The Misting Spray also contains Geranium, Bergamot (furocoumarin-free), Copaiba, Black Spruce, Orange, Lime, Sage, and Ocotea Essential Oils. Other natural ingredients include aloe vera, vanilla fruit extract, and a trace mineral complex.

The Misting Spray nourishes and refreshes the skin with 100% pure essential oils, provides an aroma that inspires confidence, is made with naturally derived, plant-based ingredients, is vegan friendly, and is formulated without alcohol, parabens, phthalates, petrochemicals, synthetic fragrances, or synthetic colorants.

The Savvy Minerals by Young Living™ Lipsticks are formulated to bring out every woman's unique and natural beauty. They have a creamy texture, which glides on smoothly, and medium coverage, which improves the appearance of lip fullness. With natural-looking, beautiful shades, these lipsticks add just the right amount of shine and color to your lips. Savvy Minerals lipsticks are made with naturally derived ingredients, including castor seed oil, sweet almond oil, candelilla wax, beeswax, and vitamin E. They are also cruelty-free and were formulated without parabens, phthalates, petrochemicals, bismuth, talc, synthetic fragrances, or synthetic colorants.

Age Refining Technology (ART®) Line: Refreshing Toner

Young Living Age Refining Technology (ART®) products were created to offer an essential oil-infused line of products for those looking to slow down or reduce the signs of aging skin. These products contain only naturally derived ingredients and therapeutic-grade essential oils. They spoil your skin without the artificial ingredients and irritating chemicals contained in many skin care products. This line is a perfect solution for those who want a natural product to support healthy-looking skin and a more youthful appearance.

In a matter of seconds, a simple sweep of the ART® Refreshing Toner can help balance your skin's pH levels, reduce the appearance of pores, and completely remove any residual particles that cleansing may have missed. The perfect blend of essential oils and natural ingredients will leave your face clean, toned, and refreshed. It was formulated with Peppermint, Royal Hawaiian™ Sandalwood, Frankincense, Lavender, Lemon, and Melissa Essential Oils. Other natural ingredients include witch hazel water, betaine from plant juice, orchid flower extract, aloe juice, and green tea extract. If you love the Refreshing Toner, be sure to check out the other products in the ART® line, including the Gentle Cleanser, Light Moisturizer, Renewal Serum, and more.

For the Gentlemen

Although most of the previous research looked at the toxicity of female personal care products, some recent studies specifically evaluated the dangers of male care products. On average, men use six grooming or beauty products a day, containing an average of 85 chemicals, most of these identical to the ones found in female beauty cosmetics.[348] It's time to spoil our men by giving them non-toxic personal care and grooming products that are not only formulated without toxins but are full of natural ingredients that have been used for centuries.

Throughout history, a variety of plants have been used all over the world to boost healthy male performance, including ashwagandha, long jack, fenugreek, tribulus terrestris, epimedium, muira puama, and sesame seeds. Now we have the technology to research these botanicals to understand the effects they have on the human body.

Ashwagandha belongs to the Solanaceae family and is also known as "Indian Ginseng" or "Winter Cherry." In Ayurvedic medicine, it is called "The Rejuvenator" and is one of the most important herbs in those teachings. But ashwagandha is also found in Southeast Asian and African folk medicine. It is an adaptogen, which means that it is a natural substance considered to help the body adapt to stress.

Ashwagandha exerts a normalizing effect upon physical, chemical, or biological stresses without adverse effects. Numerous studies have shown the many positive effects Ashwagandha can have on the human body.[349] Ashwagandha is regarded as an adaptogenic tonic, an aphrodisiac, a stress-reliever, a diuretic, an astringent, and a thermogenic and stimulating substance. The name for the root comes from its horse-like ("ashwa") smell ("gandha"). Folklore states that after consuming ashwagandha, you will have the power of a horse. It has shown to improve cognitive functions, such as memory, executive function, sustained attention, and information-processing speed.[350]

It was also reported that ashwagandha supplementation is associated with significant increases in muscle mass and strength[351] while decreasing muscle injuries.[352] There was significant improvement of maximum oxygen uptake (VO2 max), metabolic equivalents METS (an estimate of how many calories are burned during physical activity), and time to exhaustion on a treadmill in elite cyclists.[353] Researchers using a special formulation of Ashwagandha, KSM-66, also demonstrated enhanced cardio-respiratory endurance and improved quality-of-life (QOL) in healthy athletic adults.[354]

Ashwagandha has been extensively researched for various sex-related effects in men. In addition to significantly improving blood hormone levels, it also demonstrated a 167% increase in sperm count, a 53% increase in semen volume, and a 57% increase in sperm motility.[355] Treatment with ashwagandha resulted in a decrease in stress, improved the level of antioxidants, and improved overall semen quality in a significant number of previously infertile male participants.

The treatment resulted in pregnancy in the partners of 14% of the patients.[356] Several authors concluded that because it decreases stress levels, improves sperm count and motility, and regulates reproductive hormone levels, ashwagandha improves male fertility.[357] Women can benefit from this supplement as well. One study demonstrated significant improvement in arousal, lubrication, orgasms, satisfaction, and the number of successful sexual encounters.[358]

Eurycoma longifolia, also known as tongkat ali or "long jack", is a popular libido-increasing herbal medicine native to Asian countries. It has a long history as one of the well-known folk medicines for aphrodisiac effects. Studies showed that it can significantly increase episodes of penile reflexes and erections, and that long jack is a potent stimulator of sexual arousal.[359,360,361] A review of multiple studies revealed a remarkable association between the use of long jack and the efficacy in the treatment of male sexual disorders in seven of eleven studies.[362]

This natural compound also showed to have positive effects on overall testosterone levels and semen quality in men.[363] Semen analyses showed significant improvements in regards to higher semen volumes, sperm concentrations, the percentage of normal sperm morphology, and sperm motility (ability to move). As a result, 14.7% of the study participants reported spontaneous pregnancies with their partners.[364] In addition, it was mentioned that high doses of long jack over time displayed beneficial effects on athletic endurance performance and physiological responses.[365]

Fenugreek (Trigonella foenum-graecum Linn.) is considered as one of the oldest medicinal plants, and its many health-promoting effects have been cited in both Ayurvedic and traditional Chinese medicine.[366] It is commonly used to control sugar, fat, and cholesterol levels[367,368] and to support antioxidant, liver protective, anti-inflammatory, antibacterial, antifungal, antiulcer, and anticarcinogenic effects on the human body.[369] Fenugreek increased the levels of free testosterone by 98.7% compared to the baseline 8 weeks earlier.[370]

Despite the fact that fenugreek is an estrogenic plant, research has demonstrated a significant positive effect on male libido and on maintaining normal healthy testosterone levels.[371] But these effects were not just isolated findings in males. Other studies showed that fenugreek use also increased free testosterone and estrogen levels as well as sexual desire and arousal in woman compared with the female placebo group. The results indicate that fenugreek can be used for increasing sexual arousal and desire in women.[372]

In ancient medicine, tribulus terrestris has been used for its diuretic, tonic, and aphrodisiac properties. Nowadays, tribulus is mostly consumed by athletes and bodybuilders because it supposedly increases testosterone. While animal studies displayed a significant increase in blood testosterone levels after tribulus administration, this effect was mostly noted in humans when it was combined with other supplements.

However, because tribulus causes nitric oxide release, which acts by opening blood vessels including those in the genitals, tribulus can have aphrodisiac properties independent of the testosterone level.[373] Other studies were able to show a statistically reliable increased anaerobic muscular power and anaerobic glycolytic power (energy from the breakdown of sugar), i.e. better athletic performance.[374]

Epimedium (Epimedium brevicornum), also called "horny goat weed" or "Yin Yang Huo," has been consumed for erectile dysfunction in traditional Chinese medicine for many centuries. The name horny goat weed was used by ancient Chinese goat herders because they notice increased sexual activity of the goats after the animals ate the leaves of this plant.

Today's medical gold standard for treatment of such problems are phosphodiesterase type 5 (PDE5) inhibitors which include what is known as the "little blue pill." They dilate (open) blood vessels, including those in the genitals, through several ways, like increasing nitric oxide, a potent vasodilator (dilator of blood vessels). Hence the erectile function promoting effect of these medical drugs. Epimedium contains a natural substance that acts as PDE5 inhibitor and therefore mimics the effects of the drugs.

In fact, we should look at this the other way around: The pharmaceutical industry mimicked the effects of epimedium when creating the synthetic analogs of that plant. The active ingredient of horny goat weed is icariin, a flavonol glycoside which acts as weak to moderate PDE5 inhibitor.[375] Drug maker Pfizer sued pharmaceutical company Lilly to try to prevent them from selling their similar drug. The courts dismissed the lawsuit on the grounds that "prior art" existed in the form of epimedium and that the claims of erection-enhancing effects of natural PDE5 inhibitors had been used for a long time.

The medical literature summarizes the broad therapeutic capabilities, especially for enhancing reproductive function, and also describes the osteo-protective, neuro-protective, cardio-protective, anti-inflammatory, immune-protective, and anti-cancer properties of icariin.[376] One study also showed that icariin can decrease depressive symptoms and reduce alcohol consumption.[377] But overall, epimedium/icariin is mostly used these days for its beneficial effects on reproductive organs and increased levels of testosterone.[378]

Muira puama (Ptychopetalum olacoides), also called "potency wood", is actually the best-known Amazonian folk medicine for increasing libido and erectile function.[379] It acts as a nerve stimulant to heighten receptiveness to sexual stimuli as well as physical sensation of sex.[380] In one study with 262 men reporting poor sexual desire, 62% reported improvements with muira puama supplementation.[381]

But women have also shown to benefit from muira puama. In combination with gingko biloba, it improved frequency of sexual desires, sexual intercourse, and sexual fantasies, as well as satisfaction with sex life, intensity of sexual desires, excitement of fantasies, ability to reach orgasm, and intensity of orgasm.[382] Most scientific studies have been done in combination with other supplements.

Also noteworthy is that at least normal-dose and short-term use of pure ashwagandha, long jack, and tribulus did not show up as doping when measured in athletes.[383,384,385] However, one anti-doping study reported an incident where a tribulus supplement was contaminated with a banned steroid.[386]

Another doping case, in 2016, looked at a testosterone-boosting supplement used by two mountain bikers and found that a combination of tribulus terrestris, eurycoma longifolia, epimedium grandiflorum, and fenugreek with other ingredients resulted in a doping charge. This highlights the fact that only supplements from a trusted, high-quality source should be used by professional athletes, and that athletes need to know about the type and the amount of ingredients in their natural products.

PowerGize™

PowerGize™ uses exotic ingredients to help support manly activities. Inspire your inner athlete with this awesome product. This essential oil infused supplement is specially formulated to help individuals of all ages boost stamina and performance. With natural botanicals from around the world, PowerGize™ helps sustain energy levels, increase muscle size and strength, enhance tone, accelerate recovery, and support mental and physical vibrancy and vitality when used in addition to physical activity. PowerGize™ promotes overall well-being and hormonal health.

This formulation contains Blue Spruce, Goldenrod, and Cassia Essential Oils. The other ingredients are ashwagandha root extract, longjack root powder, fenugreek seed extract, epimedium leaf powder, desert hyacinth (Cistanche tubulosa) root powder, tribulus fruit/leaf extract, muira puama bark powder, zinc, magnesium, and vitamin B6. PowerGize™ uses KSM-66, a premium ashwagandha root extract, which is touted for its properties that support immunity, mental clarity, concentration, and alertness. KSM-66's custom formula helps support the healthy male reproductive system.

Shutran™ Products: Shave Cream, 3-in-1 Men's Wash, Aftershave Lotion

Shutran™ products contain a powerful blend specially formulated for men to boost feelings of masculinity and confidence. The individual oils in Shutran™ have typically been used for centuries to support healthy manly activities. These products contain the Shutran™ Essential Oil blend, which includes Idaho Blue Spruce, Ocotea, Ylang Ylang, Hinoki, Coriander, Davana/Artemisia, Lavender, Cedarwood, Lemon, and Northern Lights Black Spruce Essential Oils.

Depending on the type of product, other ingredients such as aloe vera, ucuuba nut oil, zinc oxide, olive fruit oil, vitamin E, mango and cocoa butter, grapeseed oil, sugar cane extract, safflower seed oil, green tea extract, and bamboo extract have been added. The Shutran™ bath and body care line includes body wash, bar soap, shave cream, aftershave lotion, and beard oil.

Made with pure essential oils and moisturizing botanicals, the Shutran™ Shave Cream delivers an incredibly close, smooth shave. This luxurious shave cream provides a frictionless glide to reduce razor burn and nicks. In addition to the Shutran™ Essential Oil blend, it contains Tea Tree Essential Oil.

Specifically formulated for men, the Shutran™ 3-in-1 Men's Wash gives you a powerful clean that doesn't strip your skin of moisture. Don't crowd your shower shelf with lots of bottles. Shutran™ 3-in-1 Men's Wash has everything you need, so you can get on with your day and handle business. It cleanses your face, hair, and body in one easy step. Created specifically for men and infused with Young Living's rich, woodsy Shutran™ Essential Oil blend, this unique essential oil body wash will leave you feeling confident and bold. It is 100% plant-based with naturally derived ingredients, vegan-friendly, and also dermatologist tested and hypoallergenic. Shutran™ 3-in-1 Men's Wash was formulated without sulfates, parabens, phthalates, petrochemicals, animal-derived ingredients, synthetic fragrances, or synthetic colorants.

Feel as good as your shave looks with refreshing Shutran™ Aftershave Lotion. This 100% plant-based aftershave soothes, freshens, and calms skin after you've roughed it up while shaving. This aftershave won't dry out your skin and is perfectly moisturizing. Plus, application is a breeze. Shutran™ Aftershave Lotion isn't greasy and absorbs quickly into skin, providing a light cooling sensation as it restores moisture. It's the perfect shaving companion to the Shutran™ Shave Cream. Shutran™ Aftershave Lotion offers a little piece of feel-good luxury to the final step of your routine, since the vegan-friendly formula was made without parabens, EDTA, phthalates, petrochemicals, animal-derived ingredients, synthetic fragrances, or artificial colorants.

Bonus Suggestion: Doctor Oli's Hair Spray

Since some essential oils have been registered as dietary supplements by Young Living, making function-structure claims by citing the according references in the scientific literature are permitted (at least in the U.S.) when talking about essential oils or blends containing such dietary supplement essential oils.

Studies have shown that some single essential oils like lavender, rosemary, thyme, cedarwood, and peppermint, as well as some essential oil blends have been used for centuries to support healthy hair growth.

One study evaluated the topical application of a blend of essential oils including thyme, rosemary, lavender, and cedarwood in a mixture of carrier oils (jojoba and grapeseed), which was then massaged daily into the scalps of the study participants. This was compared to a placebo group using only the carrier oils.

The results showed that the application of the full mix containing these four essential oils resulted in significantly better hair growth compared to the placebo solution (44% vs. 15%).[387] The use of these essential oils was also safe, without any side effects.

In another study, the essential oil of Chamaecyparis obtusa, also called Hinoki (a cypress-like conifer tree native to Northeast Asia), promoted hair growth by activating Vascular Endothelial Growth Factor (VEGF),[388] a hair growth regulating gene. The use of Carthamus tinctorius L (safflower) florets also showed the same activating effect on the VEGF and Keratinocyte Growth Factor (KGF) genes, stimulating the hair bulbs to grow hair.[389] Similar effects could be shown by using Geranium sibiricum extract.[390]

Yet another very interesting study compared peppermint essential oil to normal saline, jojoba oil, and the most frequently used hair growth promoting pharmaceutical drug. They measured not only the activation of hair promoting genes, thickness of the scalp, increase in hair follicle numbers and hair follicle depth, but also the biomarkers for enhanced hair growth.

The results showed that peppermint essential oil was superior to all other groups in all the measurements.[391] The same study also noted that peppermint essential oil was absolutely non-toxic. And lastly, another study compared lavender essential oil to normal saline, jojoba oils, and the same medical drug as used in the previous study. The results clearly demonstrated the superiority of the non-toxic lavender essential oil in all the measurements as well.[392] It has been shown to take around six months to see a significant difference when using essential oils to support healthy hair growth.[393]

Here's my suggestion of a mix to support healthy and gorgeous hair: Take an eight-ounce glass spray bottle and fill it 80% with water. Then add 30 to 40 drops of each of the following Young Living Essential Oils: Peppermint, Cedarwood, Lavender, Thyme, Rosemary, Cypress, Hinoki, Copaiba, Geranium, and Helichrysum. Store the mix in your fridge, and apply it one to three times a day by spraying a couple spritzes into the roots of your hair and massaging it into your scalp. Make sure to shake the bottle first! Since the solution will be cold, it will have a very refreshing effect. Do this for at least six months.

Note: None of the statements made about any of Young Living's products have been evaluated by the Food and Drug Administration. Young Living products are not intended to diagnose, treat, cure, or prevent any disease.

Most of the product information and text describing Young Living products is directly from Young Living Essential Oils, LC, and can be found online at youngliving.com

Mister™, SclarEssence™, KidScents®, ART®, Savvy Minerals by Young Living™, PowerGize™, and Shutran™ are trademarks of Young Living Essential Oils, LC.

Royal Hawaiian™ Sandalwood is a trademark of Jawmin, LLC.

Month 8 Shopping Lists:

For the Ladies

Product Name	Item Number	PV
Foundation Powder-Savvy Minerals by Young Living™	Various	44
Misting Spray-Savvy Minerals by Young Living™	21397	15
ART® Refreshing Toner	5360	24.75
Lipstick -Savvy Minerals by Young Living™	Various	22.75
	Total PV:	106.5
Bonus Essential Oil: SclarEssence™		
For Your Kiddo: KidScents® Lotion		

For the Gentlemen

Product Name	Item Number	PV
Shutran™ Shave Cream	5157	20.25
Shutran™ 3-in-1 Men's Wash	20483	32
Shutran™ Aftershave Lotion	5710	26.75
PowerGize™	4748	30.5
	Total PV:	109.5
Bonus Essential Oil: Mister™		
For Your Kiddo: KidScents® Lotion		

Month 8 ER Points Earning Rate: 20%	
Rewards Points Earned this Month:	~21
Cumulative Reward Points:	~143

References:

[344] The Health Risks of Hidden Heavy Metals in Face Makeup. https:// environmentaldefence.ca/report/report-heavy-metal-hazard-the-health-risks-of-hidden-heavy-metals-in-face-makeup/.

[345] Agency for Toxic Substances and Disease Registry. Toxic Substances Portal. Propylene Glycol. https://www.atsdr.cdc.gov/substances/ toxsubstance.asp?toxid=240.

[346] U.S. Food and Drug Administration: "Trade Secrets" Ingredients. www.fda. gov/cosmetics/labeling/ucm414211.htm.

[347] U.S. Food and Drug Administration: Product Testing. www.fda.gov/ cosmetics/scienceresearch/producttesting/default.htm.

[348] Environmental Working Group. Skin Deep Cosmetics Database. Exposures add up – Survey results. www.ewg.org/skindeep/2004/06/15/exposures-add-up-survey-results/#.W4w9b-hKiUl.

[349] An Overview on Ashwagandha: A Rasayana (Rejuvenator) of Ayurveda. Afr J Tradit Complement Altern Med. 2011; 8(5 Suppl): 208–213. doi: 10.4314/ajtcam.v8i5S.9.

[350] Efficacy and Safety of Ashwagandha (Withania somnifera (L.) Dunal) Root Extract in Improving Memory and Cognitive Functions. J Diet Suppl. 2017 Nov 2;14(6):599-612. doi: 10.1080/19390211.2017.1284970.

[351] Examining the effect of Withania somnifera supplementation on muscle strength and recovery: a randomized controlled trial. J Int Soc Sports Nutr. 2015; 12: 43. doi: 10.1186/s12970-015-0104-9.

[352] Examining the effect of Withania somnifera supplementation on muscle strength and recovery: a randomized controlled trial. J Int Soc Sports Nutr. 2015 Nov 25;12:43. doi: 10.1186/s12970-015-0104-9.

[353] Effects of eight-week supplementation of Ashwagandha on cardiorespiratory endurance in elite Indian cyclists. J Ayurveda Integr Med. 2012 Oct-Dec; 3(4): 209–214. doi: 10.4103/0975-9476.104444.

[354] Efficacy of Ashwagandha (Withania somnifera [L.] Dunal) in improving cardiorespiratory endurance in healthy athletic adults. Ayu. 2015 Jan-Mar;36(1):63-8. doi: 10.4103/0974-8520.169002.

[355] Clinical Evaluation of the Spermatogenic Activity of the Root Extract of Ashwagandha (Withania somnifera) in Oligospermic Males. A Pilot Study. Evid Based Complement Alternat Med. 2013; 2013: 571420. doi: 10.1155/2013/571420.

[356] Withania somnifera Improves Semen Quality in Stress-Related Male Fertility. Evid Based Complement Alternat Med. 2011; 2011: 576962. doi: 10.1093/ecam/nep138.

[357] Role of Withania somnifera (Ashwagandha) in the management of male infertility. Reprod Biomed Online. 2018 Mar;36(3):311-326. doi: 10.1016/j. rbmo.2017.11.007.

[358] Efficacy and Safety of Ashwagandha (Withania somnifera) Root Extract in Improving Sexual Function in Women: A Pilot Study. Biomed Res Int. 2015;

2015: 284154. doi: 10.1155/2015/284154.

[359] Evaluation of the potency activity of aphrodisiac in Eurycoma longifolia Jack. Phytother Res. 2001 Aug;15(5):435-6. PMID: 11507738.

[360] Eurycoma longifolia Jack enhances libido in sexually experienced male rats. Exp Anim. 1997 Oct;46(4):287-90. PMID: 9353636.

[361] Efficacy of Tongkat Ali (Eurycoma longifolia) on erectile function improvement: systematic review and meta-analysis of randomized controlled trials. Complement Ther Med. 2015 Oct;23(5):693-8. doi: 10.1016/j. ctim.2015.07.009.

[362] Eurycoma Longifolia as a potential adoptogen of male sexual health: a systematic review on clinical studies. Chin J Nat Med. 2017 Jan;15(1):71-80. doi: 10.1016/S1875-5364(17)30010-9.

[363] Standardised water-soluble extract of Eurycoma longifolia, Tongkat ali, as testosterone booster for managing men with late-onset hypogonadism? Andrologia. 2012 May;44 Suppl 1:226-30. doi: 10.1111/j.1439-0272.2011.01168.x.

[364] Eurycoma longifolia Jack in managing idiopathic male infertility. Asian J Androl. 2010 May; 12(3): 376–380. doi: 10.1038/aja.2010.7.

[365] Review Ergogenic Effect of long jack, Eurycoma Longifolia. Pharmacogn Rev. 2016 Jul-Dec; 10(20): 139–142. doi: 10.4103/0973-7847.194041.

[366] A small plant with big benefits: Fenugreek (Trigonella foenum-graecum Linn.) for disease prevention and health promotion. Mol Nutr Food Res. 2017 Jun;61(6). doi: 10.1002/mnfr.201600950.

[367] The potential of fenugreek (Trigonella foenum-graecum) as a functional food and nutraceutical and its effects on glycemia and lipidemia. J Med Food. 2011 Dec;14(12):1485-9. doi: 10.1089/jmf.2011.0002.

[368] New legume sources as therapeutic agents. Br J Nutr. 2002 Dec;88 Suppl 3:S287-92. DOI: 10.1079/BJN2002719.

[369] Pharmacological effects of Trigonella foenum-graecum L. in health and disease. Pharm Biol. 2014 Feb;52(2):243-54. doi: 10.3109/13880209.2013.826247.

[370] Beneficial effects of fenugreek glycoside supplementation in male subjects during resistance training: A randomized controlled pilot study. Journal of Sport and Health Science Volume 5, Issue 2, June 2016, Pages 176-182. doi. org/10.1016/j.jshs.2014.09.005.

[371] Physiological aspects of male libido enhanced by standardized Trigonella foenum-graecum extract and mineral formulation. Phytother Res. 2011 Sep;25(9):1294-300. doi: 10.1002/ptr.3360.

[372] Influence of a Specialized Trigonella foenum-graecum Seed Extract (Libifem), on Testosterone, Estradiol and Sexual Function in Healthy Menstruating Women, a Randomised Placebo Controlled Study. Phytother Res. 2015 Aug;29(8):1123-30. doi: 10.1002/ptr.5355.

[373] A systematic review on the herbal extract Tribulus terrestris and the roots of its putative aphrodisiac and performance enhancing effect. J Diet Suppl. 2014 Mar;11(1):64-79. doi: 10.3109/19390211.2014.887602.

[374] The influence of the Tribulus terrestris extract on the parameters of the functional preparedness and athletes' organism homeostasis. Fiziol Zh. 2009;55(5):89-96. PMID: 20095389.

[375] Erectogenic and neurotrophic effects of icariin, a purified extract of horny goat weed (Epimedium spp.) in vitro and in vivo. J Sex Med. 2010 Apr;7(4 Pt 1):1518-28. doi: 10.1111/j.1743-6109.2009.01699.x.

[376] Anti-Cancer Properties of the Naturally Occurring Aphrodisiacs: Icariin and Its Derivatives. Front Pharmacol. 2016 Jun 29;7:191. doi: 10.3389/fphar.2016.00191.

[377] An open-label pilot study of icariin for co-morbid bipolar and alcohol use disorder. Am J Drug Alcohol Abuse. 2016 Mar;42(2):162-7. doi: 10.3109/00952990.2015.1114118.

[378] The testosterone mimetic properties of icariin. Asian J Androl. 2006 Sep;8(5):601-5. DOI: 10.1111/j.1745-7262.2006.00197.x.

[379] Asian herbals and aphrodisiacs used for managing ED. Transl Androl Urol. 2017 Apr; 6(2): 167–175. doi: 10.21037/tau.2017.04.04.

[380] Yohimbine vs. Muira puama in the treatment of erectile dysfunction. The American Journal of Natural Medicine, Nov 1994, Vol. 1, No. 3, Page 8-9.

381 A review of plant-derived and herbal approaches to the treatment of sexual dysfunctions. J Sex Marital Ther. 2003 May-Jun;29(3):185-205. DOI: 10.1080/00926230390155096.

[382] Effects of Herbal vX on libido and sexual activity in premenopausal and postmenopausal women. Adv Ther. 2000 Sep-Oct;17(5):255-62. PMID: 11186145.

[383] Banned Substances Control Group. KSM-66 Ashwagandha Is Now Bscg Certified Drug Free.

[384] Supplementation of Eurycoma longifolia Jack Extract for 6 Weeks Does Not Affect Urinary Testosterone: Epitestosterone Ratio, Liver and Renal Functions in Male Recreational Athletes. Int J Prev Med. 2014 Jun; 5(6): 728–733. PMID: 25013692.

[385] Short term impact of Tribulus terrestris intake on doping control analysis of endogenous steroids. Forensic Sci Int. 2008 Jun 10;178(1):e7-10. doi: 10.1016/j.forsciint.2008.01.003.

[386] Insights into Supplements with Tribulus Terrestris used by Athletes. J Hum Kinet. 2014 Jul 8;41:99-105. doi: 10.2478/hukin-2014-0037.

[387] Randomized Trial of Aromatherapy: Successful Treatment for Alopecia Areata. Arch Dermatol. 1999;135(5):603. doi:10-1001/pubs.Arch Dermatol.-ISSN-0003-987x-135-5-dlt0599.

[388] The essential oils of Chamaecyparis obtusa promote hair growth through the induction of vascular endothelial growth factor gene. Fitoterapia. 2010 Jan;81(1):17-24. doi: 10.1016/j.fitote.2009.06.016.

[389] Hair growth-promoting effect of Carthamus tinctorius floret extract. Phytother Res. 2014 Jul;28(7):1030-6. doi: 10.1002/ptr.5100.

[390] Hair growth-promoting effect of Geranium sibiricum extract in human

dermal papilla cells and C57BL/6 mice. BMC Complement Altern Med. 2017 Feb 13;17(1):109. doi: 10.1186/s12906-017-1624-4.

[391] Peppermint Oil Promotes Hair Growth without Toxic Signs. Toxicol Res. 2014 Dec; 30(4): 297–304. doi: 10.5487/TR.2014.30.4.297.

[392] Hair Growth-Promoting Effects of Lavender Oil in C57BL/6 Mice. Toxicol Res. 2016 Apr;32(2):103-8. doi: 10.5487/TR.2016.32.2.103.

[393] Rosemary oil vs minoxidil 2% for the treatment of androgenetic alopecia: a randomized comparative trial. Skinmed. 2015 Jan-Feb;13(1):15-21. PMID: 25842469.

CHAPTER 12

Month 9: The Great Outdoors

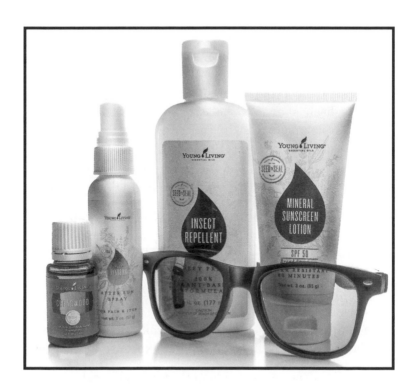

Many of us love to be outside, which often means dealing with the sun or bugs or both. Sun exposure can be beneficial and harmful at the same time, depending on intensity, time, and skin type. But all of these factors can be influenced by sun-protecting products. The sun produces ultraviolet (UV) radiation, which has three subcategories of rays/ wavelengths: UVA, UVB, and UVC.[394] UVA wavelengths account for the majority of sun radiation reaching the earth (and are also the type of radiation used in tanning beds). UVA radiation deeply penetrates the skin and induces profound alterations of the skin's tissue, playing a key role in photo-aging and photo-carcinogenesis.[395]

UVB radiation mostly affects the superficial skin layers and is the main cause of sunburns and skin cancers. It has the potential to damage the DNA of skin cells, creating dangerous mutations which can lead to a variety of skin cancers. In contrast, UVA is hardly absorbed into the DNA, but its high potential for free radical generation in the skin explains its role in the aging of skin.[396] Nevertheless, UVA has also been shown to be carcinogenic and contributes to the development of skin cancers.[397] Lastly, UVC rays typically do not make it through the atmosphere/ozone layer to reach the earth and therefore have no effect (unless the skin is exposed to artificially produced UVC radiation).

Young Living has created a variety of outdoor products formulated without toxins, including a sunscreen which protects against both UVA and UVB wavelengths. By combining safe, natural minerals with healthy skin supporting essential oils, Young Living revolutionized the sunscreen market with a reef safe product. I also want to mention that proper protection from sunlight includes sunglasses, which reduce direct light exposure to the eyes.

A variety of studies looking at the toxic chemicals found in sunscreens and their effect on the human hormone system, and therefore fertility, concluded that the negative effects on testosterone and estrogen levels might be disastrous for couples who wish to have children.[398] Who would have guessed that the use of commercially available sunscreens could be a reason for decreased human fertility? To better understand these issues, and other problems such as allergic skin reactions, inhalation injury, and carcinogenic potential, let's take a closer look at the types of sunscreens typically used.

Sunscreens on the market use three types of ingredients to protect skin from UV rays: chemical, mineral, or some form of nanotechnology-improved filters.

The most common sunscreens on the market contain chemical filters and are certainly the worst since they contain synthetic toxins, usually two to six of the following active ingredients: oxybenzone, avobenzone, octisalate, octocrylene, homosalate, and octinoxate. In the late 1970s, the FDA grandfathered the use of chemical ingredients in sunscreens and did not review their potential hazards for human safety. The most worrisome of these chemicals is oxybenzone, also called benzophenone-3 or BP3, which was added to nearly 65% of non-mineral sunscreens, according to the EWG's 2018 sunscreen database.

The American Contact Dermatitis Society (ACDS) called this group of compounds "the allergens of the year" in 2014. BP3 is an endocrine disruptor and causes low testosterone in males and endometriosis in women.[399,400] The reproductive toxicity resulting in altered birth weights of babies should alert women not to use oxybenzone-containing sunscreens while pregnant.[401] Even after giving birth, women should restrain themselves from using such sunscreens, as 85% of breast milk samples contain these toxic chemical filters.[402]

It is also extremely worrisome that these toxic endocrine disruptors have a negative effect on the thyroid gland as well as the hypothalamic–pituitary–gonadal axis.[403,404] This means that they interfere with normal metabolism, stress responses, hormonal feedback loops, and reproductive systems.

Environmentally, oxybenzone has been shown to produce a variety of toxic reactions in coral and fish ranging from reef bleaching to killing fish.[405] Knowing all of this, it seems logical that we would avoid the use of chemical filter-based sunscreens at any price especially when swimming in our oceans. However, they are still the most frequently sold sunscreen products on the market today.

Look at the so-called "inactive ingredients" too, especially the preservative methylisothiazolinone (MIT), which was 2013's ACDS "allergen of the year." Studies have clearly shown the skin allergy potential of this chemical, and researchers as well as physicians called methylisothiazolinone-related contact allergy an alarmingly fast-growing epidemic in need of urgent action.[406,407,408]

Mineral sunscreens use zinc oxide and/or titanium dioxide. The safety of mineral filter-based sunscreens, especially those based on zinc oxide, has been well established.[409] They are stable and do not break down under sun exposure. They also do not penetrate the skin or end up in the bloodstream. Zinc oxide sunscreens protect against both UVA and UVB radiation and are the sunscreens of choice listed in the Sunscreen Database of the EWG.

The downside of zinc oxide-based sunscreens is the appearance of "white marks" on the skin when being applied. In order to solve this problem many manufacturers use nanotechnology to minimize the size of the zinc (or titanium) particles resulting in better absorption of the minerals into the upper skin layers.[410] While many claim that sunscreens using nanoparticles are harmless, one particular study showed that increased amounts of nano-formulated zinc were found in the blood and urine in humans after a five-day application of sunscreen containing ZnO nanoparticles (and more in females than in males).[411] Since the scientific world is not yet clear on whether nanoparticles can cause damage to either humans or the environment, it might be prudent to avoid such new and exciting technologies until more research is available.

The Sun Protection Factor, or SPF, was introduced in 1974 to give a measure of how much of the burning radiation reaches the skin's layers. For example, applying an "SPF 10" sunscreen means that a person could stay out in the sun 10 times longer without being burned. The ingredients mostly block UVB and not UVA rays (which I mentioned earlier are also known to be carcinogenic). An SPF of 10 blocks 90% of UVB radiation, SPF 15 blocks 93%, SPF 30 blocks 97%, SPF 50 blocks 98%, and finally an SPF of 100 blocks 99%.[412]

As you can see, there is not a large difference in the UVB blocking capacities of sunscreens with higher SPFs. In fact, many specialists believe that the false security perceived by sunbathers has led to increased tanning times without increased protection - and higher skin cancer rates.[413,414] Also noteworthy: studies showed that most people do not apply enough sunscreen, which drastically decreases the UVB blocking capabilities of the products.[415]

Mineral Sunscreen Lotion

Young Living's mineral sunscreens are different from other sunscreens on the market. They are non-nano zinc oxide-based products, formulated without toxins and infused with 100% pure essential oils and other naturally derived plant- and mineral-based ingredients. This product will protect the skin from both UVA and UVB radiation.

Both Mineral Sunscreen Lotions (SPF 10 or 50) have been formulated without avobenzone, oxybenzone, retinyl palmitate, parabens, phthalates, petrochemicals, PABA and 1,4-dioxane, UV chemical absorbers, artificial colors, or synthetic fragrances. The Mineral Sunscreen Lotion SPF 50 is a great choice for sun protection. It contains skin-friendly ingredients such as non-nano zinc oxide and sunflower oil, as well as Helichrysum, Lavender, Carrot Seed, Myrrh, Ylang Ylang, and Frankincense Essential Oils. This sunscreen helps to prevent sunburn for all skin types, including sensitive skin. It is water and sweat resistant up to 80 minutes. Best of all, it is completely reef safe! Don't use toxic chemicals on your skin which kill reefs and marine life... use Young Living's powerful Mineral Sunscreen Lotion.

LavaDerm™ After-Sun Spray

The market for after-sun care products has steadily increased. Studies established the potential wound healing properties of a variety of natural plants such as aloe vera or lavender,[416,417] so many after-sun lotions, gels, or sprays contain some extracts of these plants.

After any sun exposure, soothe, moisturize, and rejuvenate your skin. I recommend Young Living's LavaDerm™ After-Sun Spray. Using menthol from mint, this spray soothes and cools the skin, providing immediate relief from the effects of outdoor activity. Plus, its moisturizing qualities from ingredients such as aloe and Lavender and Helichrysum Essential Oils help prevent peeling while leaving skin feeling soft and smooth instead of tacky or sticky. With a vegan-friendly formula made without alcohol, synthetic fragrances, or synthetic colorants, LavaDerm™ After-Sun Spray is ready for the whole family to use at the beach, on a hike, or during any outdoor playtime. It is the perfect after-sun care product.

Insect Repellent

Depending on your geographical location and the time of year, insect repellents may be an important tool to be able to really enjoy outdoor activities. According to the WHO, the mosquito is the deadliest of all animals.[418] When outdoors, you should protect yourself and your family from any potential disease-carrying insects like mosquitos. Insect repellents from natural sources, like the scents of certain plants or smoke from fires, have been used for thousands of years.

Over the last century or so, natural insect repellents were commercially replaced with toxic chemicals. In the 1940s, dichloro-diphenyl-trichloroethane (DDT) was developed as the first modern synthetic insecticide. Some of you may remember the 1947 jingle created by PennSalt Chemicals which sang "DDT is good for me-e-e!" while advertising this highly toxic chemical. In 1972, the EPA issued a cancellation order for DDT based on its adverse environmental effects, such as those to wildlife, and its potential human health risks.[419] A recent review of several studies concluded that the most effective application of insect repellents is a combination of topical application of either N-diethyl-3-methylbenzamide (also known as N, N-diethyl-m-toluamide, or DEET) or picaridin, and permethrin-impregnated or other pyrethroid-impregnated clothing over topically treated skin.[420]

However, concerns have been raised over the risk of adverse toxic effects of DEET products, especially in young children and pregnant or breast-feeding women.[421] DEET-based repellents have been associated with toxic encephalopathy including seizures, numbness, and behavioral changes,[422,423] the potential to develop nasal cancers from inhalation contact,[424] compromised immune system,[425] cardiovascular toxicity and respiratory

146

distress,[426] and severe allergic reactions.[427] DEET-induced encephalopathy in children was not only caused by ingestion or repeated and extensive application of the repellents, but also occurred after brief exposure to DEET.[428]

The authors of this study suggested that repellents containing DEET are not safe when applied to children's skin and should be avoided. Even more bad news: mosquitos and other insects can develop an insensitivity once pre-exposed to DEET which then decreases the repellency of DEET-based insect repellents.[429] Since the potential toxicity of DEET is high, less toxic preparations should be substituted for DEET-containing repellents whenever possible.

I found several reports describing natural alternatives to DEET or other chemical-based repellents while searching the scientific and medical literature. A 2005 study investigated 38 essential oils in regards to their potency in repelling mosquitos and identified that citronella, clove, and patchouli essential oils were the most effective. In fact, the best protection in this study came from clove essential oil.[430] Another study investigated the efficacy of DEET, picaridin, tea tree essential oil, peppermint essential oil, and citronella essential oil on repelling kissing bugs and concluded that citronella essential oil was superior to any of the other solutions.[431]

Citronella was also tested against DEET in preventing mosquito bites. Both protected against bites, but DEET worked longer compared to citronella. However, when vanillin (from vanilla extract) was added to the citronella essential oil, the complete mix was found to last at least three hours.[432] A different study looked at the combination of lemongrass and xanthoxylum (citrus-like shrubs and trees) essential oils and vanillin and found that this combination was superior in complete protection time against mosquitos compared to DEET.[433] Several authors concluded that the addition of vanillin to either single essential oils or blends significantly increased the complete repellency time[434,435] and therefore this mixture represents a valid natural alternative for those who would like to avoid chemicals while enjoying the outdoors annoyance-free.

Young Living's Insect Repellent is made with 100% naturally derived, plant-based ingredients and essential oils traditionally recommended for their bug-repellent properties. It is formulated without DEET, parabens, fillers, phthalates, petrochemicals, animal-derived ingredients, synthetic preservatives, synthetic fragrances, or synthetic colorants. It was tested to repel mosquitoes, ticks, and fleas naturally with 99% active ingredients plus one percent vitamin E.

This insect repellent is hypoallergenic and appropriate for use in children and people with sensitive skin. Ingredients include Citronella, Lemongrass, Rosemary, Geranium, Spearmint, Thyme, and Clove Essential Oils. Ditch any chemical-containing insect repellents and start using Young Living's natural Insect Repellent.

Cedarwood Essential Oil

Cedarwood (Cedrus atlantica) Essential Oil has a woodsy, warm, balsamic aroma that creates a relaxing, calming, and comforting atmosphere when diffused. Products made from cedarwood have long been used to protect against a variety of insects including regular ants, fire ants, ticks, and moths.[436,437] However, one study showed that the essential oil of cedarwood alone failed to protect from mosquitos.[438]

Because of the calming and comforting atmosphere it creates, diffusion of Cedarwood Essential Oil could be the perfect method to support a healthy, annoyance-free sleep in the great outdoors. It also has skin-cleansing properties and acts as a natural deodorizer, all good benefits for an active, nature-filled lifestyle. In addition to these effects, Cedarwood Essential Oil helps to maintain the appearance of youthful skin and healthy-looking hair. Enjoy the outdoors annoyance-free with Cedarwood Essential Oil alone or blended with other essential oils such as Citronella, Rosemary, Tea Tree, Myrtle, Clove, or Lemongrass.

Month 9 Shopping List:

Product Name	Item Number	PV
Mineral Sunscreen Lotion SPF 50	24137	29.75
LavaDerm™ After-Sun Spray	20673	24.75
Insect Repellent	20701	38.75
Cedarwood Essential Oil	3509	11.5
	Total PV:	106.5
Bonus Essential Oil: Citronella		
For Your Kiddo: KidScents® Owie™ Essential Oil		
Month 9 ER Points Earning Rate: 20%		
Rewards Points Earned this Month:		~21.3
Cumulative Reward Points:		~164.53

Note: None of the statements made about any of Young Living's products have been evaluated by the Food and Drug Administration. Young Living products are not intended to diagnose, treat, cure, or prevent any disease.

Most of the product information and text describing Young Living products is directly from Young Living Essential Oils, LC, and can be found online at youngliving.com

KidScents®, Owie™, and LavaDerm™ are trademarks of Young Living Essential Oils, LC.

References:

[394] UV Radiation and the Skin. Int J Mol Sci. 2013 Jun; 14(6): 12222–12248. doi: 10.3390/ijms140612222.

[395] New insights in photoaging, UVA induced damage and skin types. Exp Dermatol. 2014 Oct;23 Suppl 1:7-12. doi: 10.1111/exd.12388.

[396] Photocarcinogenesis: UVA vs UVB. Methods Enzymol. 2000;319:359-66. PMID: 10907526.

[397] Ultraviolet A-induced DNA damage: role in skin cancer. Bull Acad Natl Med. 2014 Feb;198(2):273-95. PMID: 26263704.

[398] Environmental Working Group. The Trouble With Ingredients in Sunscreens. https://www.ewg.org/sunscreen/report/the-trouble-with-sunscreen-chemicals/#.W66RuWhKiUk.

[399] Serum testosterone concentrations and urinary bisphenol A, benzophenone-3, triclosan, and paraben levels in male and female children and adolescents: NHANES 2011-2012. Environ Health Perspect 124:1898-1904; http://dx.doi.org/10.1289/EHP150.

[400] Urinary Concentrations of Benzophenone-type UV Filters in US Women and Their Association with Endometriosis. Environ Sci Technol. 2012 Apr 17; 46(8): 4624–4632. doi: 10.1021/es204415a.

[401] Exposure to benzophenone-3 and reproductive toxicity: A systematic review of human and animal studies. Reprod Toxicol. 2017 Oct;73:175-183. doi: 10.1016/j.reprotox.2017.08.015.

[402] Exposure patterns of UV filters, fragrances, parabens, phthalates, organochlor pesticides, PBDEs, and PCBs in human milk: correlation of UV filters with use of cosmetics. Chemosphere. 2010 Nov;81(10):1171-83. doi: 10.1016/j.chemosphere.2010.09.079.

[403] Recent Advances on Endocrine Disrupting Effects of UV Filters. Int J Environ Res Public Health. 2016 Aug; 13(8): 782. doi: 10.3390/ijerph13080782.

[404] Endocrine activity and developmental toxicity of cosmetic UV filters—An update. Toxicology. 2004;205:113–122. doi: 10.1016/j.tox.2004.06.043.

[405] Dermatological and environmental toxicological impact of the sunscreen ingredient oxybenzone/benzophenone-3. J Cosmet Dermatol. 2018 Feb;17(1):15-19. doi: 10.1111/jocd.12449.

[406] Methylisothiazolinone contact allergy--growing epidemic. Contact Dermatitis. 2013 Nov;69(5):271-5. doi: 10.1111/cod.12149.

[407] Methylchloroisothiazolinone and methylisothiazolinone contact allergy: an occupational perspective. Contact Dermatitis. 2015 Jun;72(6):381-6. doi: 10.1111/cod.12379.

[408] Epidemic of Isothiazolinone Allergy in North America: Prevalence Data From the North American Contact Dermatitis Group, 2013-2014. Dermatitis. 2017 May/Jun;28(3):204-209. doi: 10.1097/DER.0000000000000288.

[409] Risk assessment of zinc oxide, a cosmetic ingredient used as a UV filter of sunscreens. J Toxicol Environ Health B Crit Rev. 2017;20(3):155-182. doi:

10.1080/10937404.2017.1290516.

[410] The Advancing of Zinc Oxide Nanoparticles for Biomedical Applications. Bioinorg Chem Appl. 2018; 2018: 1062562. doi: 10.1155/2018/1062562.

[411] Small Amounts of Zinc from Zinc Oxide Particles in Sunscreens Applied Outdoors Are Absorbed through Human Skin. Toxicological Sciences 118(1):140-9. DOI: 10.1093/toxsci/kfq243.

[412] Skin Cancer Foundation. https://www.skincancer.org/prevention/sun-protection/sunscreen/sunscreens-explained.

[413] Environmental Working Group's Guide to Sunscreens. What's Wrong With High SPF?

[414] Sunscreen use and intentional exposure to ultraviolet A and B radiation: a double blind randomized trial using personal dosimeters. Br J Cancer. 2000 Nov; 83(9): 1243–1248. doi: 10.1054/bjoc.2000.1429.

[415] Sunscreen use at Danish beaches and how to improve coverage. Dan Med J. 2018 Apr;65(4). pii: B5476. PMID: 29619938.

[416] The efficacy of aloe vera used for burn wound healing: a systematic review. Burns. 2007 Sep;33(6):713-8. DOI: 10.1016/j.burns.2006.10.384.

[417] Antioxidant and wound healing activity of Lavandula aspic L. ointment. J Tissue Viability. 2016 Nov;25(4):193-200. doi: 10.1016/j.jtv.2016.10.002.

[418] World Health Organization WHO. Mosquito-borne diseases. Mosquitoes cause millions of deaths every year. http://www.who.int/neglected_diseases/vector_ecology/mosquito-borne-diseases/en/.

[419] Environmental Protection Agency EPA. https://www.epa.gov/ingredients-used-pesticide-products/ddt-brief-history-and-status.

[420] Chemical and Plant-Based Insect Repellents: Efficacy, Safety, and Toxicity. Wilderness Environ Med. 2016 Mar;27(1):153-63. doi: 10.1016/j.wem.2015.11.007.

[421] DEET-based insect repellents: safety implications for children and pregnant and lactating women. CMAJ. 2003 Aug 5;169(3):209-12. PMID: 12900480.

[422] Toxic encephalopathy associated with use of DEET insect repellents: a case analysis of its toxicity in children. Hum Exp Toxicol. 2001 Jan;20(1):8-14. DOI: 10.1191/096032701676731093.

[423] Topical use of DEET insect repellent as a cause of severe encephalopathy in a healthy adult male. Acad Emerg Med. 1999 Dec;6(12):1295-7. PMID: 10609933.

[424] Genotoxicity studies on permethrin, DEET and diazinon in primary human nasal mucosal cells. Eur Arch Otorhinolaryngol. 2002 Mar;259(3):150-3. PMID: 12003267.

[425] N,N,-Diethyl-m-Toluamide (DEET) Suppresses Humoral Immunological Function in B6C3F1 Mice. TOXICOLOGICAL SCIENCES 108(1), 110–123 (2009) doi:10.1093/toxsci/kfp001.

[426] Insect repellent (N,N-diethyl-m-toluamide) cardiovascular toxicity in an adult. Ann Pharmacother. 1993 Mar;27(3):289-93. DOI:

10.1177/106002809302700305.

[427] Severe allergic reaction to diethyltoluamide (DEET) containing insect repellent. Allergy Asthma Clin Immunol. 2014; 10(Suppl 2): A30. doi: 10.1186/1710-1492-10-S2-A30.

[428] Toxic encephalopathy associated with use of DEET insect repellents: a case analysis of its toxicity in children. Hum Exp Toxicol. 2001 Jan;20(1):8-14. DOI: 10.1191/096032701676731093.

[429] Aedes aegypti mosquitoes exhibit decreased repellency by DEET following previous exposure. PLoS One. 2013;8(2):e54438. doi: 10.1371/journal.pone.0054438.

[430] Comparative repellency of 38 essential oils against mosquito bites. Phytother Res. 2005 Apr;19(4):303-9. DOI: 10.1002/ptr.1637.

[431] Repellency of DEET, picaridin, and three essential oils to Triatoma rubida (Hemiptera: Reduviidae: Triatominae). J Med Entomol. 2013 May;50(3):664-7. PMID: 23802464.

[432] Effectiveness of citronella preparations in preventing mosquito bites: systematic review of controlled laboratory experimental studies. Trop Med Int Health. 2011 Jul;16(7):802-10. doi: 10.1111/j.1365-3156.2011.02781.x.

[433] Toxicity and synergic repellency of plant essential oil mixtures with vanillin against Aedes aegypti (Diptera: Culicidae). J Med Entomol. 2012 Jul;49(4):876-85. PMID: 22897048.

[434] Repellent activity of selected essential oils against Aedes aegypti. Fitoterapia. 2007 Jul;78(5):359-64. DOI: 10.1016/j.fitote.2007.02.006.

[435] Plant-based insect repellents: a review of their efficacy, development and testing. Malar J. 2011; 10(Suppl 1): S11. doi: 10.1186/1475-2875-10-S1-S11.

[436] Bioactivity of cedarwood oil and cedrol against arthropod pests. Environ Entomol. 2014 Jun;43(3):762-6. doi: 10.1603/EN13270.

[437] Chemical Composition and Larvicidal Activities of the Himalayan Cedar, Cedrus deodara Essential Oil and Its Fractions Against the Diamondback Moth, Plutella xylostella. J Insect Sci. 2011; 11: 157. doi: 10.1673/031.011.15701.

[438] Repellency of essential oils to mosquitoes (Diptera: Culicidae). J Med Entomol. 1999 Sep;36(5):625-9. PMID: 10534958.

$\mathcal{L}$CHAPTER 13

Month 10: Treat Your Body

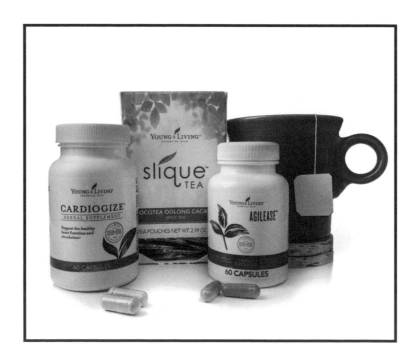

What supplements do I suggest for your monthly order? It is difficult to decide on individual recommendations for dietary supplements since each one of us has different issues and needs. However, in light of the obesity epidemic around the world and its consequences on cardiovascular disease, I decided to concentrate on products intended to support a healthy body weight and a healthy heart. In addition, because of the increase in joint and bone-related issues in both young and aging people in our society, I also wanted to address products that support healthy bones and joints.

Many people today suffer from various forms of nutritional deficiencies. These deficits are caused by food processing, bad overall nutrition, food preparation, and certain diets. In general, people do not eat enough fruits and vegetables, and instead replace these important food sources with processed and sugary foods.[439] Nutritional deficiencies in children with low fruit and vegetable consumption were twice as high as those with the usual consumption amounts.[440]

Also, low fruit and vegetable ingestion is associated with a higher incidence of cardiovascular diseases and mortality.[441,442,443] Such a lack of nutrition is also associated with neurological problems,[444] skin issues,[445] gastrointestinal diseases,[446] diabetes,[447] cancer,[448,449] and metabolic syndromes[450] including obesity.[451]

But it is not just about what you don't eat; maybe even more important is what you do eat, especially when combined with a lack of physical exercise. Today's foods are heavily treated with chemicals and preservatives from the moment they are planted. After harvest, they are commercially cleaned with chemicals, and synthetic preservatives are added to prolong expiration dates. The inclusion of sugar or equivalent sugary compounds such as high-fructose corn syrup has become a real problem as well.

In light of this nutritional transition from natural food to processed food products and high calorie sugar-rich diets over the last 30 to 40 years, many countries have witnessed the prevalence of obesity in its citizens double and even quadruple.[452] The increase of childhood obesity is reaching epidemic levels and is an especially big concern.

Childhood obesity can profoundly affect the physical health, social interactions, and emotional well-being of children, as well as their self-esteem. Childhood obesity is also associated with poor academic performance and a lower quality of life. Many co-morbid conditions like metabolic, cardiovascular, neurological, hepatic, pulmonary, renal, and orthopedic issues are also seen in association with childhood obesity.[453]

A higher intake of foods rich in flavonoids (the healthy compounds in a plant) contributes to weight maintenance in adulthood and plays a role in the prevention of obesity and its potential consequences.[454] When studying pairs of twins with different levels of flavonoid intake, a higher habitual consumption of a number of flavonoids is associated with lower fat mass independent of shared genetics and common environmental factors.[455]

Slique® Tea

Drinks known to have high flavonoid and polyphenol content are teas.[456] For example, oolong tea has demonstrated the capability to decrease body fat content and reduce body weight through improving lipid metabolism.[457] It also reduced high-fat diet-induced fat accumulation.[458] Hot oolong tea consumption was inversely associated with obesity, which means that hot tea consumers had a lower mean waist circumference and a lower Body Mass Index (BMI) compared to non-tea drinkers.[459] Hot tea consumption was also associated with beneficial biomarkers of cardiovascular disease risk and inflammation. Please note that all of this was true with consumption of hot oolong tea, but not iced oolong tea. In fact, consumption of iced tea showed just the opposite.

Interestingly enough, the activation of TRP Vanilloid (TRPV) receptors in the nerve endings of the gut and in the brain can result in an increase of satiety.[460] Both vanilla as well as incensole acetate from frankincense have shown to activate these receptors. Therefore, a beverage containing oolong tea, vanilla, frankincense, and similar ingredients would likely be beneficial for achieving and maintaining a healthy body weight.

Slique® Tea was formulated with jade oolong tea, inulin, ocotea leaf, Ecuadorian cacao powder, vanilla essential oil, 100% pure therapeutic grade frankincense powder (Boswellia sacra), and natural stevia extract. It is an exotic drink from Young Living that has been created to help support individual weight goals. This blend is rich in flavonoids, a dietary compound generally associated with helping maintain certain normal and healthy body functions. Slique® tea also contains polyphenols, which may be useful as part of a guilt-free weight-management regimen when combined with a healthy diet and physical activity. Slique® Tea is part of the Slique® line, which has many products intended to support a heathy body weight and overall wellness.

CardioGize™

There is clear evidence that the negative trends of excess body weight also lead to an increased incidence of cardiovascular diseases.[461] Occurrences of high blood pressure, stroke, heart attacks, and even dying from these conditions is clearly on the rise. In fact, cardiovascular events are still the leading cause of global mortality.[462] For the total U.S. population, heart disease has been the leading cause of death for decades, with cancer second.[463]

The risk of getting these diseases increases with poor nutrition and lack of physical activity. The question of whether dietary supplements can decrease overall morbidity (getting the disease) or mortality (dying from the disease) is still hotly debated depending on the type of dietary supplement. But there is no doubt that improving nutrition, treating the microbiome, and increasing physical exercise will have a beneficial effect.

While the overall assessment of dietary supplements is still unclear, individual supplements made from natural sources have shown positive effects on not just cardiovascular but also other type of diseases.

In 2015, an interesting report looked at the dietary supplements of selenium and coenzyme Q10 in relation to cardiovascular parameters. The authors found a better cardiac function according to echocardiography imaging, a lower concentration of a biomarker indicating lower stress of the heart muscle (lower myocardial wall tension), as well as reduction of cardiovascular mortality.[464]

Some recent studies confirm this finding and show that supplementation with a combination of selenium with coenzyme Q10 was able to lower mortality from cardiovascular events by about 50%.[465] Even after a 12-year follow-up, the mortality was still significantly reduced.[466]

The use of garlic as a medicinal compound goes back to the Sumerians, ancient Egyptians, and the ancient Greek. Ancient Chinese and Indian medicine also recommended garlic to aid a variety of conditions. Since then, garlic, and its preparations, have been widely used for prevention and treatment of cardiovascular diseases.

A wealth of medical literature supports the notion that garlic consumption has significant cardioprotective effects by lowering blood pressure, preventing atherosclerosis, reducing serum cholesterol and triglyceride, inhibiting platelet aggregation, and increasing fibrinolytic (blood clot dissolving) activity.[467,468,469,470]

Vitamin K (K for the German word Koagulation) is a vitamin typically known for its blood clotting properties. However, there are mainly two forms of this vitamin. While vitamin K1 is mostly involved with regulation of blood clotting, vitamin K2 keeps calcium in the bones and out of the blood vessels.[471,472] Vitamin K2 in the form of menaquinone, but not vitamin K1, has shown to prevent calcification of coronary blood vessels, decreasing the risk for cardiovascular problems such as heart attacks and reducing the mortality of such cardiac events by up to 50%.[473,474]

Another study revealed that vitamin K2 supplementation was associated with a 12% increase in maximal cardiac output (how much blood the heart can pump).[475] Menaquinone-7 is the preferred form of supplementation with vitamin K2 because it has a longer half-life and better tissue distribution than other vitamin K-forms.[476]

Our bones produce a substance called osteocalcin, which helps take calcium from the blood circulation and bind it to the bone. However, osteocalcin needs vitamin K2 to become fully activated and do its job. This also makes vitamin K2 a major player in bone health.[477]

CardioGize™ is a supplement that blends essential oils and a balanced combination of herbs and compounds to help support the cardiovascular system. This special product may promote a higher quality of life by supporting healthy heart function and blood circulation. It uses the proper synergistic ratio of CoQ10 and selenium. Deodorized garlic and CoQ10 provide antioxidant properties, and the vitamin K supports healthy vascular system function. CardioGize™ also includes natural folate, astragalus, dong quai, motherwort, cat's claw, cactus powder, and hawthorn berry, all used traditionally for cardiovascular support, making it a great addition to the daily herbal supplements in your routine. Other ingredients include Angelica, Cardamom, Cypress, Lavender, Helichrysum, Rosemary, and Cinnamon Bark Essential Oils. (Please consult with your doctor if you are on blood thinners.)

AgilEase™

As we age, bone and joint issues become a common problem. In most people over 55 years of age, joint issues are not isolated to a single joint.[478] The rate of reporting joint problems increases tremendously with age, from five percent for subjects aged 16-24 years, to 54% for those aged 85 years and older.[479] Knee and lower back pain are the most frequent types of joint or bone pain described by people 55 years and older. Knee pain occurs in up to 28% of this age group, and lower back pain occurs in up to 80% (and women suffer more often than men).[480,481] In the U.S., about 57% of all doctor visits are related to osteoarthritis, joint disorders, or back problems.[482]

Another big issue is osteoporosis, since it is the most common bone disease in humans. With an aging population and longer life span, osteoporosis is increasingly becoming a global epidemic.[483] Currently, it has been estimated that more than 200 million women globally are suffering from osteoporosis. According to recent statistics from the International Osteoporosis Foundation, one in three women over the age of 50 worldwide, and one in five men, will experience osteoporotic fractures in their lifetime.[484]

Annually, osteoporosis causes more than 8.9 million fractures across the globe, resulting in an osteoporotic fracture every three seconds. Among those, forearm, hip, and back fractures are almost equally represented.[485] And if someone suffers one fracture, the risk of a subsequent fracture related to osteoporosis increases by 86%.[486] Osteoporotic fractures represent a significant cause of morbidity and mortality, particularly in developed countries.[487]

Exercising regularly decreases osteoporosis, and therefore osteoporotic fractures, and increases overall joint health. It is also important to know that osteoporotic fractures are not just caused by demineralization of the bone alone, but they are also caused by the loss of muscle mass in aging people. This increases the risk of a fall with subsequent bone and joint injury. By age 70, people are expected to lose between 50% and 55% of their maximum muscle mass.[488]

Exercise will not only strengthen the bones but also help to maintain muscle mass and improve overall balance. These are all important factors in preventing injury in aging people. The right amount of joint movement is also important for younger people. The various parts of a joint including cartilage, capsule, meniscus, disc, and ligament need movement for optimal functioning and prevention of decay. In addition, regular movement and weightbearing decreases pain associated with problems in muscles, joints, and bones.[489,490]

Glucosamine is among the most sold over-the-counter supplements worldwide. Glucosamine supplementation demonstrated a chondroprotective (protection of cartilage in joints) effect in soccer players by preventing type II collagen degradation while maintaining type II collagen synthesis.[491] However, the effect was transient and disappeared after quitting glucosamine ingestion. Hyaluronic acid, another popular supplement used for joint health, has shown to reduce osteoarthritis symptoms and structural damage and delay prosthetic joint surgery.[492]

Oral supplementation with hyaluronic acid over 12 months demonstrated a reduction of joint symptoms in people under the age of 70, particularly when combined

160

with exercise. The symptoms started to improve as early as two months into supplementation.[493] While it makes a lot of sense to supplement calcium to increase bone mass, more recent studies have shown that calcium supplementation alone has a small positive effect on overall bone density.[494] The data shows a trend toward reduction in vertebral fractures and improved lasting upper limb bone density. So, calcium intake seems to have a small positive effect on bone mineral content or bone mineral density.

On the other hand, undenatured type II collagen supplementation has clearly shown to improve knee joint symptoms and to be well-tolerated.[495] Another study also showed significant improvements to joint pain, joint function, and quality of life after three months of supplementation with native type II collagen.[496]

When using natural compounds, frankincense has been shown to have beneficial effects in regards to joint pain and increased functionality after only a few days of supplementation, with no serious adverse effects.[497,498,499]

AgilEase™ is a joint health supplement that is perfect for individuals who are looking to keep up their active lifestyles by supporting joint mobility and flexibility. It can reduce acute joint discomfort and support the body's healthy response to inflammation from exercise.

Young Living formulated this product with unique and powerful ingredients such as frankincense powder, UC-II undenatured collagen, hyaluronic acid, curcuminoids from turmeric, piperidine from black pepper, calcium fructoborate from plants, and a specially formulated proprietary essential oil blend of Wintergreen, Copaiba, Clove, and Northern Lights Black Spruce. These are oils that are known for their joint health benefits. AgilEase™ is beneficial for athletes and active individuals of all ages who want to support and protect their joints and cartilage. It is a perfect companion to an active lifestyle and helps ease acute joint discomfort to improve quality of life.

Bonus Product: Master Formula™

A recent survey of over 10,000 people who use dietary supplements shows the most popular dietary supplement is fish oil, followed by multivitamin products.[500] As an alternative (or in addition) to the above-mentioned product suggestions, you could also order Young Living's Master Formula™. This product is a full spectrum, multi-nutrient complex, providing premium vitamins, minerals, and food-based nutrients to support general health and wellbeing.

By utilizing a Synergistic Suspension Isolation process (SSI Technology) the ingredients are delivered in three distinct delivery forms. Collectively, these ingredients provide a premium complex to support your body. Master Formula™ naturally supports general health and provides gut flora supporting prebiotics. Other ingredients help neutralize free radicals in the body. Master Formula™ is pre-packaged in individual daily sachets in order to make it convenient to take your vitamins on the go.

Note: None of the statements made about any of Young Living's products have been evaluated by the Food and Drug Administration. Young Living products are not intended to diagnose, treat, cure, or prevent any disease.

Most of the product information and text describing Young Living products is directly from Young Living Essential Oils, LC, and can be found online at youngliving.com

EndoFlex™ Vitality™, KidScents®, MightyZyme™, Slique®, CardioGize™, AgilEase™, and Master Formula™ are trademarks of Young Living Essential Oils, LC.

Month 10 Shopping List:

Product Name	Item Number	PV
Slique® Tea	4560	20.25
CardioGize™	21696	39.75
AgilEase™	5764	47
	Total PV:	107
Bonus Essential Oil: EndoFlex™ Vitality™		
For Your Kiddo: MightyZyme™ Chewable Tablets		
Month 10 ER Points Earning Rate: 20%		
Rewards Points Earned this Month:		~21
Cumulative Reward Points:		~185

References:

[439] Consumption of fruits and vegetables among adolescents: a multi-national comparison of eleven countries in the Eastern Mediterranean Region. Br J Nutr. 2016 Mar 28;115(6):1092-9. doi: 10.1017/S0007114515005371.

[440] Associations between low consumption of fruits and vegetables and nutritional deficiencies in Brazilian schoolchildren. Public Health Nutr. 2015 Apr;18(5):927-35. doi: 10.1017/S1368980014001244.

[441] Low consumption of fruit and vegetables and risk of chronic disease: a review of the epidemiological evidence and temporal trends among Spanish graduates. Public Health Nutr. 2011 Dec;14(12A):2309-15. doi: 10.1017/S1368980011002564.

[442] Fruit and vegetable consumption is inversely associated with blood pressure in a Mediterranean population with a high vegetable-fat intake: the Seguimiento Universidad de Navarra (SUN) Study. Br J Nutr. 2004 Aug;92(2):311-9. DOI: 10.1079/BJN20041196.

[443] Fruit and vegetable consumption and risk of cardiovascular disease: A meta-analysis of prospective cohort studies. Crit Rev Food Sci Nutr. 2017 May 24;57(8):1650-1663. doi: 10.1080/10408398.2015.1008980.

[444] Fruit and vegetable consumption and the risk of depression: A meta-analysis. Nutrition. 2016 Mar;32(3):296-302. doi: 10.1016/j.nut.2015.09.009.

[445] Diet and Dermatology. The Role of Dietary Intervention in Skin Disease. J Clin Aesthet Dermatol. 2014 Jul; 7(7): 46–51. PMID: 25053983.

446 Consumption of vegetables and fruit and the risk of inflammatory bowel disease: a meta-analysis. Eur J Gastroenterol Hepatol. 2015 Jun;27(6):623-30. doi: 10.1097/MEG.0000000000000330.

447 Fruit and vegetable consumption and risk of type 2 diabetes mellitus: a dose-response meta-analysis of prospective cohort studies. Nutr Metab Cardiovasc Dis. 2015 Feb;25(2):140-7. doi: 10.1016/j.numecd.2014.10.004.

448 Vegetables, fruit, and cancer prevention: a review. J Am Diet Assoc. 1996 Oct;96(10):1027-39. DOI: 10.1016/S0002-8223(96)00273-8.

449 Fruit, vegetable, and antioxidant intake and all-cause, cancer, and cardiovascular disease mortality in a community-dwelling population in Washington County, Maryland. Am J Epidemiol. 2004 Dec 15;160(12):1223-33. PMID: 15583375.

450 Fruit and vegetable consumption and risk of the metabolic syndrome: a meta-analysis. Public Health Nutr. 2018 Mar;21(4):756-765. doi: 10.1017/S136898001700310X.

451 Fruit and Vegetable Intake and Body Mass Index in a Large Sample of Middle-Aged Australian Men and Women. Nutrients. 2014 Jun; 6(6): 2305–2319. doi: 10.3390/nu6062305.

452 The Epidemiology of Obesity: A Big Picture. Pharmacoeconomics. 2015 Jul; 33(7): 673–689. doi: 10.1007/s40273-014-0243-x.

453 Childhood obesity: causes and consequences. J Family Med Prim Care. 2015 Apr-Jun;4(2):187-92. doi: 10.4103/2249-4863.154628.

454 Dietary flavonoid intake and weight maintenance: three prospective cohorts of 124 086 US men and women followed for up to 24 years. BMJ. 2016; 352: i17. doi: 10.1136/bmj.i17.

455 Higher dietary flavonoid intakes are associated with lower objectively measured body composition in women: evidence from discordant monozygotic twins. Am J Clin Nutr. 2017 Mar;105(3):626-634. doi: 10.3945/ajcn.116.144394.

456 Tea and flavonoids: where we are, where to go next? Am J Clin Nutr. 2013 Dec; 98(6): 1611S–1618S. doi: 10.3945/ajcn.113.059584.

457 Beneficial effects of oolong tea consumption on diet-induced overweight and obese subjects. Chin J Integr Med. 2009 Feb;15(1):34-41. doi: 10.1007/s11655-009-0034-8.

458 Aged Oolong Tea Reduces High-Fat Diet-Induced Fat Accumulation and Dyslipidemia by Regulating the AMPK/ACC Signaling Pathway. Nutrients. 2018 Feb; 10(2): 187. doi: 10.3390/nu10020187.

459 Tea consumption is inversely associated with weight status and other markers for Metabolic Syndrome in U.S. adults. Eur J Nutr. 2013 Apr; 52(3): 1039–1048. doi: 10.1007/s00394-012-0410-9.

460 Transient Receptor Potential Channels as Targets for Phytochemicals. ACS Chem Neurosci. 2014 Nov 19; 5(11): 1117–1130. doi: 10.1021/cn500094a.

461 Obesity and Cardiovascular Disease. Circ Res. 2016 May 27;118(11):1752-70. doi: 10.1161/CIRCRESAHA.115.306883.

[462] Estimating Deaths From Cardiovascular Disease: A Review of Global Methodologies of Mortality Measurement. Circulation. 2013 Feb 12; 127(6): 749–756. doi: 10.1161/CIRCULATIONAHA.112.128413.

[463] Changes in the Leading Cause of Death: Recent Patterns in Heart Disease and Cancer Mortality. NCHS Data Brief. 2016 Aug;(254):1-8. PMID: 27598767.

[464] Selenium and coenzyme Q10 interrelationship in cardiovascular diseases--A clinician's point of view. J Trace Elem Med Biol. 2015;31:157-62. doi: 10.1016/j.jtemb.2014.11.006.

[465] Supplementation with Selenium and Coenzyme Q10 Reduces Cardiovascular Mortality in Elderly with Low Selenium Status. A Secondary Analysis of a Randomised Clinical Trial. PLoS One. 2016 Jul 1;11(7):e0157541. doi: 10.1371/journal.pone.0157541.

[466] Still reduced cardiovascular mortality 12 years after supplementation with selenium and coenzyme Q10 for four years: A validation of previous 10-year follow-up results of a prospective randomized double-blind placebo-controlled trial in elderly. PLoS One. 2018 Apr 11;13(4):e0193120. doi: 10.1371/journal.pone.0193120.

[467] Garlic and Heart Disease. J Nutr. 2016 Feb;146(2):416S-421S. doi: 10.3945/jn.114.202333.

[468] A review of the cardiovascular benefits and antioxidant properties of allicin. Phytother Res. 2013 May;27(5):637-46. doi: 10.1002/ptr.4796.

[469] Garlic and cardioprotection: insights into the molecular mechanisms. Can J Physiol Pharmacol. 2013 Jun;91(6):448-58. doi: 10.1139/cjpp-2012-0315.

[470] Garlic (Allium sativum L.) and cardiovascular diseases. Bratisl Lek Listy. 2010;111(8):452-6. PMID: 21033626.

[471] High dietary menaquinone intake is associated with reduced coronary calcification. Atherosclerosis. 2009 Apr;203(2):489-93. doi: 10.1016/j. atherosclerosis.2008.07.010.

[472] Proper Calcium Use: Vitamin K2 as a Promoter of Bone and Cardiovascular Health. Integr Med (Encinitas). 2015 Feb; 14(1): 34–39. PMID: 26770129.

[473] Dietary intake of menaquinone is associated with a reduced risk of coronary heart disease: the Rotterdam Study. J Nutr. 2004 Nov;134(11):3100-5. DOI: 10.1093/jn/134.11.3100.

[474] A high menaquinone intake reduces the incidence of coronary heart disease. Nutr Metab Cardiovasc Dis. 2009 Sep;19(7):504-10. doi: 10.1016/j. numecd.2008.10.004.

[475] Oral Consumption of Vitamin K2 for 8 Weeks Associated With Increased Maximal Cardiac Output During Exercise. Altern Ther Health Med. 2017 Jul;23(4):26-32. PMID: 28646812.

[476] Menaquinone-7 Supplementation to Reduce Vascular Calcification in Patients with Coronary Artery Disease: Rationale and Study Protocol (VitaK-CAC Trial). Nutrients. 2015 Nov; 7(11): 8905–8915. doi: 10.3390/ nu7115443.

[477] Osteocalcin: the vitamin K-dependent Ca2+-binding protein of bone matrix. Haemostasis. 1986;16(3-4):258-72. DOI: 10.1159/000215298.

[478] Impact of multiple joint problems on daily living tasks in people in the community over age fifty-five. Arthritis Rheum. 2006 Oct 15;55(5):757-64. DOI: 10.1002/art.22239.

[479] Changing profile of joint disorders with age: findings from a postal survey of the population of Calderdale, West Yorkshire, United Kingdom. Ann Rheum Dis. 1992 Mar;51(3):366-71. PMID: 1533506.

[480] Knee pain and disability in the community. Br J Rheumatol. 1992 Mar;31(3):189-92. PMID: 1540789.

[481] Acute and Chronic Low Back Pain. Med Clin North Am. 2016 Jan;100(1):169-81. doi: 10.1016/j.mcna.2015.08.015.

[482] Why do patients visit their doctors? Assessing the most prevalent conditions in a defined US population. Mayo Clin Proc. 2013 Jan; 88(1): 56–67. doi: 10.1016/j.mayocp.2012.08.020.

[483] An overview and management of osteoporosis. Eur J Rheumatol. 2017 Mar; 4(1): 46–56. doi: 10.5152/eurjrheum.2016.048.

[484] International Osteoporosis Foundation. Osteoporosis - Incidence and burden. https://www.iofbonehealth.org/facts-statistics.

[485] An estimate of the worldwide prevalence and disability associated with osteoporotic fractures. Osteoporos Int. 2006 Dec;17(12):1726-33. DOI: 10.1007/s00198-006-0172-4.

[486] A meta-analysis of previous fracture and subsequent fracture risk. Bone. 2004 Aug;35(2):375-82. DOI: 10.1016/j.bone.2004.03.024.

[487] An estimate of the worldwide prevalence and disability associated with osteoporotic fractures. Osteoporos Int. 2006 Dec;17(12):1726-33. DOI: 10.1007/s00198-006-0172-4.

[488] The Role of Exercises in Osteoporotic Fracture Prevention and Current Care Gaps. Where Are We Now? Recent Updates. Rambam Maimonides Med J. 2017 Jul; 8(3): e0032. PMID: 28786812.

[489] The pain-relieving qualities of exercise in knee osteoarthritis. Open Access Rheumatol. 2013; 5: 81–91. doi: 10.2147/OARRR.S53974.

[490] The effectiveness of physiotherapy interventions for sacroiliac joint dysfunction: a systematic review. J Phys Ther Sci. 2017 Sep; 29(9): 1689-1694. doi: 10.1589/jpts.29.1689.

[491] Evaluation of the effect of glucosamine administration on biomarkers for cartilage and bone metabolism in soccer players. Int J Mol Med. 2009 Oct;24(4):487-94. PMID: 19724889.

[492] Effectiveness and utility of hyaluronic acid in osteoarthritis. Send to Clin Cases Miner Bone Metab. 2015 Jan-Apr;12(1):31-3. doi: 10.11138/ccmbm/2015.12.1.031.

[493] Oral Administration of Polymer Hyaluronic Acid Alleviates Symptoms of Knee Osteoarthritis: A Double-Blind, Placebo-Controlled Study over a 12-Month Period. ScientificWorldJournal. 2012; 2012: 167928. doi:

10.1100/2012/167928.

[494] Calcium supplementation on bone loss in postmenopausal women. Cochrane Database Syst Rev. 2004;(1):CD004526. DOI: 10.1002/14651858. CD004526.pub2.

[495] Efficacy and tolerability of an undenatured type II collagen supplement in modulating knee osteoarthritis symptoms: a multicenter randomized, double-blind, placebo-controlled study. Nutr J. 2016; 15: 14. doi: 10.1186/s12937-016-0130-8.

[496] Effects of Native Type II Collagen Treatment on Knee Osteoarthritis: A Randomized Controlled Trial. Eurasian J Med. 2016 Jun; 48(2): 95–101. doi: 10.5152/eurasianjmed.2015.15030.

[497] FlexiQule (Boswellia extract) in the supplementary management of osteoarthritis: a supplement registry. Minerva Med. 2014 Dec;105(6 Suppl 2):9-16. PMID: 26076376.

[498] A double blind, randomized, placebo controlled clinical study evaluates the early efficacy of aflapin in subjects with osteoarthritis of knee. Int J Med Sci. 2011;8(7):615-22. PMID: 22022214.

[499] Hand 'stress' arthritis in young subjects: effects of Flexiqule (pharma-standard Boswellia extract). A preliminary case report. Minerva Gastroenterol Dietol. 2015. PMID: 26492590.

[500] The most-used supplements in America right now. ConsumerLab.com Report 2015. www.newhope.com/breaking-news/most-used-supplements-america-right-now.

❧CHAPTER 14

Month 11: Baby Talk

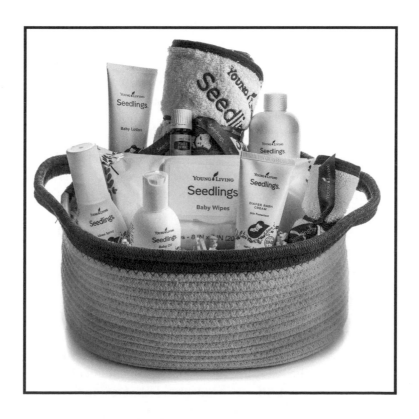

When a baby is born, it's natural that the parents look at their wonderful miracle and want only the best for this new developing human. Unfortunately, many of the commercially available products for babies and young children on the market contain toxic chemicals and endanger our most vulnerable population group.

Babies and young children are more susceptible to chemicals from personal care products than adults because a child's skin is 30% thinner and can absorb greater amounts of chemicals. The blood-brain barrier, which blocks toxins and chemicals in the blood from penetrating brain tissue, is not fully developed until a baby is six months old. And even then, many toxins will cross the blood-brain barrier leading to potential life-long damage.

Here are some toxic chemicals found in infant products: 1,4-dioxane which is used in some bubble baths and body washes; bisphenol A (BPA), which can be found in some baby bottles, water bottles and metal food containers; formaldehyde, which is used in some baby shampoos and body washes; parabens, which can be found in some baby care products; phthalates, which are used in many baby care products; polyvinyl chloride (PVC), which is found in baby toys; sodium lauryl sulfate (SLS), which is used in some baby washes and shampoos; synthetic fragrances, used in many baby personal care products; tributyl-tin (TBT), which is found in some baby diapers; and triclosan, which is found in baby soaps and washes. 1,4-dioxane and formaldehyde are both known carcinogens.

A study conducted by the EWG revealed that 82% of the tested bath products for children contained formaldehyde, 67% contained 1,4-dioxane, and 61% contained both chemicals.[501] Even baby products labelled as "gentle" or "natural" may be loaded with various toxic chemicals. Since the FDA has no authority to demand that companies test their products before they are sold, or list potentially toxic ingredients on product labels, our infants are at high risk of exposure to such chemicals.

According to the EWG, children are exposed to these dangerous chemicals every day due to personal care products alone. In an online survey of more than 3,300 parents, this organization found that the average child is exposed to 27 chemicals a day from body care products. These ingredients have not been found safe for children, including some associated with cancer, brain and nervous system damage, allergies, and hormone disruption.[502]

These chemicals are common ingredients in baby shampoos, lotions, diaper creams, sunscreens, and several other children's body care products. And babies are not just exposed to these toxins after they are born. A study revealed that 287 chemicals could be detected in umbilical cord blood, 180 of them known to cause cancer in humans or animals, 217 of them known to be toxic to the brain and nervous system, and 208 of them known to cause birth defects or abnormal development in animal tests.[503]

The EWG also mentions in the source described earlier that 82% of children are exposed every week to one or more ingredients with the potential to harm the brain and nervous system, 69% of children are exposed every week to one or more ingredients that may disrupt the hormone system, 3.6% of children are exposed to ingredients with strong data linking them to cancer, and 80% of children's products marked as gentle and non-irritating contain ingredients linked to allergies and skin or eye irritation.

A growing body of evidence shows adverse effects of endocrine disrupting chemicals on child development including fetal growth, early reproductive tract development, pubertal development, neurodevelopment, and obesity.[504] A study measuring phthalates and their metabolites in 163 infants found that phthalate exposure is widespread and that infant exposure to lotions, powders, and shampoos was significantly associated with increased urinary concentrations of monoethyl phthalate, monomethyl phthalate, and monoisobutyl phthalate.

These associations increased with the number of baby products used.[505] Phthalates are known to be endocrine disruptors and to adversely affect hormones and reproductive systems. A review found that young boys are especially at risk for low testosterone levels, cryptorchidism (one or both of the testes fail to descend from the abdomen into the scrotum during childhood development), and small genital size. Phthalates therefore have an anti-virilizing effect in infants.[506]

In regards to the quickly increasing rates of childhood and adult obesity, it was found that poor diet and a lack of exercise alone could not explain this phenomenon. So, the "obesogen hypothesis"[507] was created, and more recent research confirms that the increase of chemicals in human tissue is in fact an important factor in obesity and other diseases. To make things worse, epigenetic changes (the influence of certain proteins on the DNA) caused by chemicals make these adverse effects on body weight inheritable.

Overall, epidemiological studies in humans suggest effects of endocrine disruptors on prenatal growth, thyroid function, glucose metabolism and obesity, puberty, fertility, and on carcinogenesis mainly through epigenetic mechanisms.[508]

Obesity (including in children), diabetes, and metabolic syndromes might be inherited down through several generations.[509] One study measured epigenetic changes caused by an endocrine disrupting chemical in four generations of offspring and found these changes in all of them.[510] Several authors concluded that exposure to these toxic chemicals during the critical period of early development (pre and post-natal) created grave consequences for the health of offspring.[511] Studies showed that the average one-month-old baby is bathed four times a week, and shampooed three times a week, and therefore exposed to up to 66 chemicals weekly. Most of these babies, a whopping 78%, developed skin rashes from the toxins contained in the products.[512]

Talcum powders represent another real danger in baby care. Many cases of powder inhalation issues, even deaths, have been reported, and many household incidents associated with baby powders have been reported to poison centers.[513] A study in the 1990s found that 69% of American parents used powders regularly on their children.[514]

The use of talcum powders carries the risk of lung injury[515] and formation of ovarian cancer.[516] Over 1,000 lawsuits have now been filed regarding baby powders, mostly by women with ovarian cancer. In the past couple of years, several juries awarded these women with monetary compensation of approximately 50 to 80 million U.S. dollars.[517]

The EWG showed that 97% of bubble bath products, 95% of baby wipes, 92% of baby shampoos, and 91% of baby lotions contained so-called impurities, i.e. potentially harmful ingredients.[518] Among the chemicals found in commercially available baby wipes are formaldehyde, ethylene oxide, phenoxyethanol, parabens, methylisothiazolinone,[519] and 1,4-dioxane, all of which have shown potential toxicity, especially in infants.

Many physicians and child protection groups have called for much stricter rules and regulations when it comes to infant products. I am now asking all parents who read this to reconsider their purchases, get rid of any chemical-containing baby products, and only use those formulated without toxins.

Since we can't usually trust ingredient labels, you have to know the history and philosophy of companies who create these kinds of products. Parents should look for disclosures of what is NOT in the baby products which will help tremendously. And remember, exposure to toxic chemicals does not only occur to infants through the use of baby care products, but also from all other toxic sources in a household including artificial air fresheners, candles, household cleaners, laundry detergents, etc. Ditch as many chemicals as possible in your household to create a safe environment for your babies, children, and yourself.

With all of this in mind, Young Living created the Seedlings™ line of baby products. The soothing, plant-based formulas use infant-safe, 100% pure essential oils and are free from harmful ingredients, like lanolin, parabens, phthalates, petrochemicals, synthetic preservatives, synthetic fragrances, or synthetic colorants. Seedlings™ products are hypoallergenic, non-greasy, and dermatologist tested to give you peace of mind and leave your baby feeling snug and secure.

Seedlings™ Diaper Rash Cream

The Seedlings™ Diaper Rash Cream was created to help relieve, treat, and prevent diaper rash and is made with 100% naturally derived ingredients, including botanicals, non-nano zinc oxide, mango butter, and murumuru butter. When applied at the first sign of redness it reduces the duration and severity of diaper rash. The cream soothes on contact, protects your baby's delicate skin, and acts as a physical barrier to wetness. Seedlings™ Diaper Rash cream includes Lavender, German Chamomile, Black Spruce, English Marigold, and Helichrysum Essential Oils.

Seedlings™ Baby Lotion, Calm

The Seedlings™ Baby Lotion is a non-greasy, gentle moisturizer specially formulated for the delicate skin of an infant. It prevents dryness by soothing and moisturizing their thin skin. Seedlings™ Baby Lotion is formulated with 100% naturally derived ingredients, like coriander seed oil, bergamot seed oil (furocoumarin free), apple fruit extract, and mango, murumuru, and cocoa butters. This product also features the "Calm" Essential Oil blend, which includes Lavender, Geranium, Ylang Ylang, and English Marigold to soothe your baby with a light, calming scent and no unwanted ingredients.

Seedlings™ Baby Wash & Shampoo, Calm

The Seedlings™ Baby Wash & Shampoo is specially formulated for your infant's delicate skin and hair. This mild, gentle, tear-free formula is 100% plant-based. The natural ingredients include Lavender, Geranium, and Ylang Ylang Essential Oils, as well as coriander seed oil, bergamot seed oil (furocoumarin free), euphrasia (eyebright), and English marigold extract.

Seedlings™ Baby Wipes, Calm

The Seedlings™ Baby Wipes were formulated to provide gentle and thorough cleansing without drying your infant's delicate skin. These versatile wipes are made with a soft, thick material that can handle a variety of messes and can be used on any part of your infant's skin. This mild and gentle formula contains cleansing botanicals and is specially formulated to minimize the risk of common allergic reactions.

The natural ingredients include coriander seed oil, bergamot seed oil (furocoumarin free), apple fruit extract, soapberry fruit extract, aloe vera, English marigold extract, and witch hazel leaf extract, as well as Lavender, Geranium, and Ylang Ylang Essential Oils.

Seedlings™ Gift Bundle

If you want to avoid ordering all these Seedlings™ products individually, you can order the Seedlings™ Gift Bundle instead. It is perfect for your new nursery or a friend's baby shower. It includes Baby Wipes, Baby Oil, Baby Wash & Shampoo, Baby Lotion, Linen Spray, and Diaper Rash Cream, all part of Young Living's Seedlings™ line. Each item heavily features the soothing scent of Lavender Essential Oil to help create a calming environment for you and your baby, from bath time to bedtime and everywhere in between.

This bundle also comes with a hooded bath towel and washcloth created just for the set. Made with 100% unbleached cotton, this washcloth and bath towel are ready for bath time and help give your baby a cuddly, comfortable clean. Everything in the set comes together in an unbleached cotton rope basket.

Peace & Calming™ Essential Oil

The wonderful aroma of Peace & Calming™ Essential Oil is certainly a favorite scent among Young Living members. Peace & Calming™ Essential Oil is a gentle and sweet blend containing Ylang Ylang, Orange, Tangerine, Patchouli, and Blue Tansy Essential Oils. Diffuse this calming oil to freshen the air, especially in rooms where children play, study, or sleep. Apply to the bottoms of your family's feet as part of a bedtime ritual.

Please do not forget to dilute any essential oil prior to applying it to the feet of a baby; the skin of an infant is very thin and sensitive, and the oils are very strong. Please also note that Blue Tansy Essential Oil actually has a blue color. After applying to the skin, it will quickly change to a yellowish color and then completely disappear when it is fully absorbed into the skin. Therefore, it has the potential of staining bed linens.

Month 11 Shopping List:

Product Name	Item Number	PV
Seedlings™ Gift Bundle	20721	80.25
Peace & Calming™ Essential Oil	3398	34.75
	Total PV:	115
Bonus Essential Oil: Gentle Baby™		
For Your Kiddo: KidScents® SleepyIze™ Essential Oil		
Month 11 ER Points Earning Rate: 20%		
Rewards Points Earned this Month:		~23
Cumulative Reward Points:		~208

Note: None of the statements made about any of Young Living's products have been evaluated by the Food and Drug Administration. Young Living products are not intended to diagnose, treat, cure, or prevent any disease.

Most of the product information and text describing Young Living products is directly from Young Living Essential Oils, LC, and can be found online at youngliving.com

Gentle Baby™, KidScents®, SleepyIze™, Seedlings™, and Peace & Calming™ are registered trademarks of Young Living Essential Oils, LC.

References:

[501] Environmental Working Group. Toxic Chemicals In Kids' Bath Products. https://www.ewg.org/research/campaign-safe-cosmetics-report-toxic-chemicals-found-kids-bath-products#.W7ElvmhKiUk.

[502] Environmental Working Group. Children Exposed Daily to Personal Care Products With Chemicals Not Found Safe For Kids. https://www.ewg.org/news/news-releases/2007/11/01/children-exposed-daily-personal-care-products-chemicals-not-found-safe#.W7EBRGhKiUk.

[503] Environmental Working Group. Body Burden: The Pollution In Newborns. https://www.ewg.org/research/body-burden-pollution-newborns#.W61GjWhKiUk.

[504] Exposure to environmental endocrine disruptors and child development. Arch Pediatr Adolesc Med. 2012 Oct;166(10):952-8. PMID: 23367522.

[505] Baby care products: possible sources of infant phthalate exposure. Pediatrics. 2008 Feb;121(2):e260-8. doi: 10.1542/peds.2006-3766. DOI: 10.1542/peds.2006-3766.

[506] Possible impact of phthalates on infant reproductive health. Int J Androl. 2006 Feb;29(1):172-80; discussion 181-5. DOI: 10.1111/j.1365-2605.2005.00642.x.

[507] Chemical toxins: a hypothesis to explain the global obesity epidemic. J Altern Complement Med. 2002 Apr;8(2):185-92. DOI: 10.1089/107555302317371479.

[508] Current Knowledge on Endocrine Disrupting Chemicals (EDCs) from Animal Biology to Humans, from Pregnancy to Adulthood. Int J Mol Sci. 2018 Jun 2;19(6). pii: E1647. doi: 10.3390/ijms19061647. DOI: 10.3390/ijms19061647.

[509] Epigenetics: a molecular link between environmental factors and type 2 diabetes. Diabetes. 2009 Dec;58(12):2718-25. doi: 10.2337/db09-1003.

[510] Endocrine disruptor vinclozolin induced epigenetic transgenerational adult-onset disease. Endocrinology. 2006 Dec;147(12):5515-23. DOI: 10.1210/en.2006-0640.

[511] Childhood obesity and endocrine disrupting chemicals. Ann Pediatr Endocrinol Metab. 2017 Dec; 22(4): 219–225. doi: 10.6065/apem.2017.22.4.219.

[512] Newborn chemical exposure from over-the-counter skin care products. Clin Pediatr (Phila). 1991 May;30(5):286-9. DOI: 10.1177/000992289103000504.

[513] Inhalation of baby powder: an unappreciated hazard. BMJ 1991;302:1200-1.

[514] Baby powder use in infant skin care. Parental knowledge and determinants of powder usage. Send to Clin Pediatr (Phila). 1984 Mar;23(3):163-5. DOI: 10.1177/000992288402300306.

[515] Pulmonary talc granulomas, pulmonary fibrosis, and pulmonary hypertension resulting from intravenous injection of talc-containing drugs

intended for oral use. Proc (Bayl Univ Med Cent). 2002 Jul; 15(3): 260–261. PMID: 16333448.

[516] The Association Between Talc Use and Ovarian Cancer. Epidemiology. 2016 May; 27(3): 334–346. doi: 10.1097/EDE.0000000000000434.

[517] Latest baby powder lawsuit snares Walgreens. Crain's Chicago Business. https://www.chicagobusiness.com/article/20170302/NEWS03/170309953/chicago-baby-powder-lawsuit-snares-walgreens.

[518] Environmental Working Group Skin Deep Database. Impurities of Concern in Personal Care Products. http://www.ewg.org/skindeep/2007/02/04/impurities-of-concern-in-personal-care-products/#.W7EXUWhKiUk.

[519] Six children with allergic contact dermatitis to methylisothiazolinone in wet wipes (baby wipes). Pediatrics. 2014 Feb;133(2):e434-8. doi: 10.1542/peds.2013-1453.

⚘CHAPTER 15

Month 12: Let's Get Cookin'

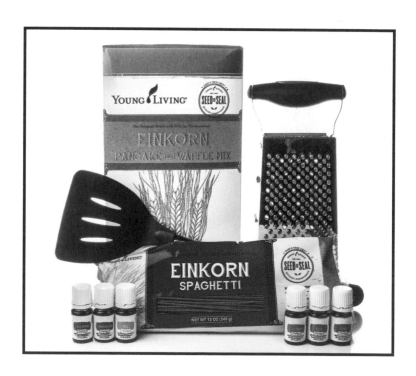

I already mentioned the importance of proper nutrition several times, but one aspect in particular deserves some more attention: whole grains. We know that the regular consumption of healthy whole grains is associated with a reduced risk of type 2 diabetes,[520] better management of obesity,[521] reduction of cardiovascular diseases (including lower cardiovascular mortality rate in the elderly),[522] a reduction in cancer occurrence,[523] and an overall reduction in chronic diseases.[524] But today's question is more about what defines a healthy whole grain product, especially since ancient versions have emerged as a great alternative to modern-day commercial hybridized grains.

Gary Young spent a lot of effort to rediscover the ancient grain we call "einkorn." During one of his travels to Egypt, he took pictures of hieroglyphics which showed people harvesting something that looked very familiar to Gary: very long stems of grains, just as he used to see and harvest in his father's fields as a young boy decades earlier. But it did not look in any way close to the wheat we see commonly today.

In 1995, Mary and Gary Young flew to Pakistan to find the Hunzakut people, famous for their longevity. The Hunza land is a mountainous valley in the Gilgit-Baltistan region of northern Pakistan. When they drove up to the Karimabad Valley, they noticed some people along the river harvesting wheat by hand.[525] That wheat looked very similar to that which Gary used to see as a boy and was depicted in the ruins of upper Egypt.

In subsequent years, he also found this grain in Anatolia, Turkey and along the Jordan River. Gary then started to cultivate it, together with his French friend Jean-Noel, on a farm in France (where it is also called "little spelt"). Today, this grain is mostly known as einkorn. Depending on the geographical location, einkorn might be called "little farro" or "fake farro." And "farro" is also sometimes used as collective term for a variety of ancient grains.

In order to avoid further confusion, I will only talk about the type of ancient wheat Gary Young cultivated in France and the U.S. for the past two decades: einkorn. Since Gary spent so much effort to bring us this ancient grain, it deserves a closer look.

As always, Gary was ahead of current research. Recent studies have demonstrated the health benefits of einkorn bread, especially the sourdough fermentation type. Einkorn has a much higher concentration of carotenoid levels than found in modern wheats. It was also revealed that einkorn bread has anti-inflammatory effects.[526] Furthermore, this ancient type of wheat has some dietary advantages over current day's wheats.

Einkorn includes a better concentration of several antioxidant compounds such as carotenoids, tocols, conjugated polyphenols, alkylresorcinols, and phytosterols as well as low β-amylase and lipoxygenase activities (which both limit antioxidant degradation during processing). It was therefore concluded that einkorn flour has excellent nutritional properties, superior to those of other wheat varieties.[527]

Gary mentioned to me early on that the gluten content of einkorn was less than $1/10^{th}$ of the gluten content of modern wheat, and that in his experience, it could sometimes be tolerated even by people with gluten sensitivities or celiac disease. This statement seems to be supported by at least one study,[528] however the scientific community has not yet reached a conclusion on this topic.[529] Of course, every person is different and will need to carefully evaluate their own tolerance of einkorn if suffering from one of these issues.

Gluten sensitivities are a big problem in today's population. Celiac disease is an inherited condition characterized by a specific genetic genotype (HLA-DQ2 and HLA-DQ8 genes) and autoantibodies.[530] It only affects up to one percent of the world population,[531] while wheat allergies affect about four percent.[532] Non-celiac gluten sensitivity (NCGS) is a recently recognized form of the gluten-related disorders.[533] Many people claiming to suffer NCGS issues have reported a massive improvement in their symptoms after eliminating gluten from their diet. Current research estimates the incidence of NCGS to be up to 13%, but practitioners in the field report rates as high as 30%, about one third of the population.[534]

Symptoms of gluten sensitivity include bloating, abdominal discomfort, nausea, diarrhea, constipation, alternating bowel habits, irritable bowel syndrome, flatulence, and gastrointestinal reflux. Systemic manifestations include tiredness, headache, fibromyalgia-like joint/muscle pain, leg or arm numbness, a 'foggy mind,' dermatitis, skin rash, depression, anxiety, and anemia.[535] For those on a gluten-free diet, the ingestion of prolamine peptide (gliadin), derived from wheat, rye, barley, oats, bulgur wheat, and any hybrids of these grains, should be avoided. They should be replaced with rice, corn, potato-derived products, and grains such as amaranth, buckwheat, manioc, fonio, teff, millet, quinoa, and sorghum.

Gary Young was convinced that the low gluten content and low reactivity in NCGS people was because einkorn (triticum monococcum) was the only non-hybridized or non-genetically modified grain among modern wheat, barley, bulgur wheat, durum wheat, graham, kamut, rye, semolina, spelt, and triticale. And research proved him right. Einkorn lacked toxicity even in the cells of celiac disease patients due to its low gluten content of around seven to nine percent.[536] Einkorn is suggested as a good choice when re-introducing alternative grains to patients with gluten sensitivities.[537]

Don't forget that most commercial crops are heavily sprayed and treated with pesticides and herbicides such as glyphosate. When we ingest these commercial grains, we also get a nasty portion of glyphosate into our body. In fact, it could be shown that glyphosate by itself is responsible for some of the so-called gluten sensitivity.[538]

Let's learn some more about Gary's beloved ancient grain. Einkorn has a diploid genome of fourteen chromosomes (two complements of seven chromosomes).[539] Over time, it hybridized with other grasses and formed grains with sets of 28 and 42 chromosomes, two or three genomes respectively. Tetraploid wheats, such as emmer and durum, contain four sets of seven chromosomes, and are derived from the hybridization between two diploid wild grasses.

Hexaploid wheats, containing six sets of seven chromosomes each, have evolved since biblical times, resulting in the modern-day wheat with a total of 42 chromosomes.[540] The fact that einkorn only has a total of 14 chromosomes means it has an unaltered gluten structure and gliadin genes which may be why it does not affect those with gluten sensitivities, intolerances, or even celiac disease, as much as other forms of wheat.[541,542] Whole grain einkorn is also two and a half times richer in protein and three times higher in antioxidants compared to modern-day commercial wheat.[543]

Ditch any modern-day wheat, switch to einkorn as a known healthy alternative, and refresh your body with this wonderful ancient nutrition-rich grain. And to make it easy for you, Young Living now offers an entire line of einkorn products. I suggest that you start with Gary's True Grit® Einkorn Pancake & Waffle Mix and Gary's True Grit® Einkorn Spaghetti, but be sure to check out the other products in this line as well.

Vitality™ Essential Oils

Since some essential oils have been registered as dietary supplements by Young Living, function-structure claims citing the appropriate references in scientific literature are permitted, at least in the U.S.

Cooking with essential oils is easy once you know the basics. All of the essential oils mentioned below are well-suited for healthy cooking. They are part of Young Living's Vitality™ line of oils, which labels essential oils as dietary supplements and allows for their internal ingestion. Overall, the positive properties of these herbs and spices are well-known and well-documented, some for thousands of years.

In addition to enjoying their wellness supporting effects, you can use these oils to enhance the flavors of a variety of foods. Be aware that essential oils may evaporate when cooking at high temperatures. I recommend adding a small amount of the oils while the cooked food is decreasing in temperature. Essential oils are very powerful substances in potency and flavor.

When first learning to cook with essential oils, I recommend inserting a toothpick into the bottle and touch that to the food you want to flavor. With this method, you get less than one full drop of essential oil which can sometime be overpowering for a dish. Start with less and add more. Be aware that it only takes one or two drops of an essential oil to flavor an entire dish.

It is best not to apply the essential oils directly onto meat, fish, or vegetables, because essential oils absorb so quickly that it is very difficult to avoid higher concentrations in one place while having none in other areas. Taking a bite that has a lot of an herb or spice essential oil can lead to bitterness or unpleasant flavors. I recommend mixing up a marinade, my recipe is at the end of this chapter, or

184

blending the oils with something like mustard so they can be easily applied evenly on meat, fish, or vegetables.

Thyme Vitality™ Essential Oil

The wellness benefits of thyme have been known for centuries.[544] Like many other essential oils, it has a very good antioxidant capacity.[545] And thyme essential oil has shown to have a calming effect on certain genes and some compounds released within the body, which supports overall wellness.[546] I like to add a drop of Thyme Vitality™ Essential Oil to vegetable soups or stocks.

Rosemary Vitality™ Essential Oil

The excellent role rosemary oil plays in supporting healthy brain activity is well established,[547,548,549,550] and it has proven to support the calmness of humans.[551] It can also be used in the bedroom to support healthy restful sleep.[552] Rosemary and its support of a healthy metabolism made this plant one of the regular ingredients in many of the Mediterranean foods known to support longevity.[553] Try adding a drop of Rosemary Vitality™ Essential Oil to the next beef pot roast you make.

Dill Vitality™ Essential Oil

Dill is a well-known herbal culinary addition to the kitchen. It has a long history in folk and Ayurvedic medicine, where it was mostly taken to support a healthy stomach and gut due its calming effects on these organs.[554] When used, it has a supporting effect on healthy triglyceride, lipid, and cholesterol levels.[555,556] The effect on cholesterol is due to dill mimicking the basic mechanism of well-known cholesterol reducers in the medical and pharmacological world.[557]

I mention this because if you use a lot of dill in your kitchen, you want to make sure to supplement your body with dietary products that contain CoEnzyme Q10, because the same mechanism also blocks the biosynthesis of this important co-enzyme. In addition, dill has also shown to support healthy sugar levels.[558,559] Due to all these effects of dill, this herbal plant has a supportive effect on overall cardiovascular wellness.[560] Add a drop or two of Dill Vitality™ Essential Oil to your dips, sauces, or even hummus.

Basil Vitality™ Essential Oil

More than 60 varieties of basil have been identified around the world, among them "Holy Basil" with its long tradition of use in folk medicine around the world. In Ayurvedic medicine, this herb is also called the "Elixir of Life."[561] It has shown to have a supportive effect on metabolism (fat and sugar), optimal stress levels, strong brain function, and healthy blood pressure.[562] Basil essential oil has also shown to have excellent antioxidant properties[563] and healthy blood sugar supporting activity.[564]

It is also interesting to know that the use of basil in your kitchen might not only be limited to culinary applications. It can also be used to clean surfaces and support healthy suppression of common foodborne microbes.[565] For that same reason, I mix one drop of Basil Vitality™ Essential Oil into my homemade salad dressing before eating the greens. And one more bonus: basil essential oil is also known for its healthy skin promoting properties.[566]

Black Pepper Vitality™ Essential Oil

Black pepper has long been known to boost nutrient absorption and support healthy gastrointestinal functionality.[567] Dietary piperine, the main active ingredient of black pepper, favorably stimulates digestive enzymes of the pancreas, enhances the healthy digestive capacity, and supports healthy gastrointestinal food transit times.[568]

Black pepper is known to be part of a group of essential oils that all have a supporting effect on brain health, specifically the neurons in the brain.[569] It's also a good antioxidant, like basically all essential oils, and has shown to support a healthy immune system.[570] However, black pepper can interact with some medications by either prolonging or shortening their action, essentially changing their effectiveness.[571]

I personally like to use Black Pepper Vitality™ Essential Oil in connection with my exercise regimen. Why? Because black pepper essential oil has shown to promote beneficial energy metabolism during exercise by regulating carbohydrate/fat metabolism and redox signals.[572] Piperine also has a supporting effect on healthy body fat levels as well as healthy hormone balance.[573] It has also been shown that black pepper, in combination with curcumin, can support healthy muscles when taken before and after workouts.[574] Add a drop of Black Pepper Vitality™ Essential Oil to your NingXia Red for a super boost of energy.

Cinnamon Bark Vitality™ Essential Oil

Finally, let's take a closer look at cinnamon essential oil. Cinnamon, with its exotic flavor and aroma, is a key ingredient in every kitchen. Its use has been documented for almost 5,000 years, as it was used in Ancient China, by the Romans, as well as by the ancient Egyptians. It is also mentioned multiple times in the Bible. Cinnamon can be either taken from the leaves or bark of cinnamon trees, but the essential oil made from the bark is typically more potent than the one from the leaves. It is not the same as Cassia Essential Oil, which is typically obtained by distilling the bark of another tree in the cinnamon family.

Cinnamon has been called "mystical"[575] because of its plentiful wellness-supporting effects. Several studies showed that cinnamon has a very positive effect on supporting healthy sugar and fat levels in the blood.[576,577] The benefits to blood sugar levels seem to come from insulin mimetic and insulin sensitizing action of this spice.[578] Cinnamon has a supporting effect on healthy blood pressure[579] and a healthy heart.[580]

Another study described the beneficial effects of cinnamon for people with bad breath.[581] There might be a reason why Cinnamon Bark Vitality™ Essential Oil is part of Young Living's Thieves® toothpastes.

The fact that Cinnamon Essential Oil is part of the Thieves® Essential Oil blend, contained in all of Young Living's cleaning products, makes a lot of sense after reviewing the scientific literature on this spice. There are so many ways we use Cinnamon Bark Vitality™ Essential Oil. It is great in your morning coffee or tea, but you can also add it to many sweet bread recipes and baked treats.

Doctor Oli's BBQ Marinade

Many of us barbeque and grill on a regular basis. The downside of this type of cooking is the potential for the creation of carcinogenic hetero-cyclic amines (HCAs) and polycyclic aromatic hydrocarbons (PAHs).[582] These toxic byproducts of cooking meat or fish at high temperatures can damage the lining of the gut.[583] One way to prevent their occurrence is to cook or grill slowly at lower temperatures.

Another way to support healthy grilling is to use certain plants, fruits, herbs, spices, and essential oils.[584,585,586,587,588] Studies showed that some of these were able to reduce the occurrence of HCA's by up to 94%.[589,590] (Please note that a large majority of these studies did not use essential oils for that purpose, so it cannot be concluded that the essential oil of a plant would do the same compared to other preparations of the plants, spices, herbs, or fruits.)

With all of that information in mind, I present to you Doctor Oli's BBQ Marinade. Although the ingredient ideas came from the research for cooking meat while preventing HCAs and PAHs, this marinade is also delicious when added to vegetables.

Take several tablespoons of yellow mustard (the amount depends on how much will be grilled) and sprinkle in crushed, dried rosemary. Then add one drop of each of the following essential oils (Young Living Vitality™ line only, of course): Rosemary, Oregano, Marjoram, Basil, Clove, Ginger, Black Pepper, Lemongrass, and Thyme. Then, add 5 drops of Lemon Vitality™ Essential Oil. Mix well and apply to the meat, fish, or vegetables. Let it all marinate for about 15 minutes before putting it on the grill. Try to grill at lower temperatures, and be aware that more well-done meat typically has a higher content of the toxic byproducts HCAs and PAHs.

Happy grilling!

Note: None of the statements made about any of Young Living's products have been evaluated by the Food and Drug Administration. Young Living products are not intended to diagnose, treat, cure, or prevent any disease.

Most of the product information and text describing Young Living products is directly from Young Living Essential Oils, LC, and can be found online at youngliving.com

Vitality™, KidScents®, TummyGize™, and Gary's True Grit® are trademarks of Young Living Essential Oils, LC.

Month 12 Shopping List:

Product Name	Item Number	PV
Gary's True Grit® Einkorn Pancake & Waffle Mix	5300	4.25
Gary's True Grit® Einkorn Spaghetti	5301	3
Thyme Vitality™ Essential Oil	5597	14.5
Rosemary Vitality™ Essential Oil	5629	7.75
Dill Vitality™ Essential Oil	5622	16.25
Basil Vitality™ Essential Oil	5583	11
Black Pepper Vitality™ Essential Oil	5617	19.25
Cinnamon Bark Vitality™ Essential Oil	5585	24.75
Total PV:		100.75
Bonus Essential Oil: Oregano Vitality™		
For Your Kiddo: KidScents® TummyGize™ Essential Oil		
Month 12 ER Points Earning Rate: 20%		
Rewards Points Earned this Month:		~21
Cumulative Reward Points:		~229

References:

[520] Dietary substitutions for refined carbohydrate that show promise for reducing risk of type 2 diabetes in men and women. J Nutr. 145:159–163. DOI: 10.3945/jn.114.195149.

[521] Whole grain intake in relation to body weight: from epidemiological evidence to clinical trials. Nutr Metab Cardiovasc Dis. 21:901–908. DOI: 10.1016/j.numecd.2011.07.003.

[522] Cereal grains and coronary heart disease. Eur J Clin Nutr. 56:1–14. DOI: 10.1038/sj.ejcn.1601283.

[523] Whole grain intake and cancer: a review of the literature. Nutr Cancer. 1995;24(3):221-9. DOI: 10.1080/01635589509514411.

[534] Wholegrain cereals and bread: a duet of the Mediterranean diet for the prevention of chronic diseases. Public Health Nutr. 14:2316–2322. DOI:

10.1017/S1368980011002576.

[525] Ancient Einkorn. Today's Staff of Life. D. Gary Young. 2014 Young Living Essential Oils. ISBN #978-0-9905100-0-0.

[526] Integrated Evaluation of the Potential Health Benefits of Einkorn-Based Breads. Nutrients. 2017 Nov; 9(11): 1232. doi: 10.3390/nu9111232.

[527] Nutritional properties of einkorn wheat (Triticum monococcum L.). J Sci Food Agric. 2014 Mar 15;94(4):601-12. doi: 10.1002/jsfa.6382.

[528] Lack of intestinal mucosal toxicity of Triticum monococcum in celiac disease patients. Scand J Gastroenterol. 2006 Nov;41(11):1305-11.

[529] Triticum monococcum in patients with celiac disease: a phase II open study on safety of prolonged daily administration. Eur J Nutr. 2015 Sep;54(6):1027-9. doi: 10.1007/s00394-015-0892-3.

[530] Celiac Disease and Nonceliac Gluten Sensitivity: A Review. JAMA. 2017 Aug 15;318(7):647-656. doi: 10.1001/jama.2017.9730.

[531] Celiac disease: prevalence, diagnosis, pathogenesis and treatment. World J Gastroenterol. 2012 Nov 14;18(42):6036-59. doi: 10.3748/wjg.v18. i42.6036.

[532] Spectrum of gluten-related disorders: consensus on new nomenclature and classification. BMC Med. 2012 Feb 7;10:13. doi: 10.1186/1741-7015-10-13.

[533] World epidemiology of non-celiac gluten sensitivity. Minerva Gastroenterol Dietol. 2017 Mar;63(1):5-15. doi: 10.23736/S1121-421X.16.02338-2.

[534] Perlmutter David. Gluten Sensitivity – Challenged by a New Study? https:// www.drperlmutter.com/gluten-sensitivity-challenged-new-study/.

[535] An Italian prospective multicenter survey on patients suspected of having non-celiac gluten sensitivity. BMC Med. 2014 May 23;12:85. doi: 10.1186/1741-7015-12-85.

[536] Lack of intestinal mucosal toxicity of Triticum monococcum in celiac disease patients. Scand J Gastroenterol. 2006 Nov;41(11):1305-11. DOI: 10.1080/00365520600699983.

[537] Non-celiac gluten sensitivity: Time for sifting the grain. World J Gastroenterol. 2015 Jul 21; 21(27): 8221–8226. doi: 10.3748/wjg.v21. i27.8221.

[538] Glyphosate, pathways to modern diseases II: Celiac sprue and gluten intolerance. Interdiscip Toxicol. 2013 Dec; 6(4): 159–184. doi: 10.2478/intox-2013-0026.

[539] Domestication of Plants in the Old World: The Origin and Spread of Cultivated Plants in West Asia, Europe, and the Nile Valley; 3rd ed. Oxford University Press; 2000. p. 38.

[540] Plant Evolution and the Origin of Crop Species. CABI Publishing; 2004. pp. 313.

[541] Re-discovering ancient wheat varieties as functional foods. J Tradit Complement Med. 2015 Jul; 5(3): 138–143. doi: 10.1016/j.

jtcme.2015.02.004.

[542] Mapping of gluten T-cell epitopes in the bread wheat ancestors: implications for celiac disease. Gastroenterology. 2005 Feb;128(2):393-401. PMID: 15685550.

[543] Ancient Einkorn. Today's Staff of Life. The Einkorn Solution. D. Gary Young. 2014 Young Living Essential Oils. ISBN #978-0-9905100-0-0. p. 73.

[544] Thymol, thyme, and other plant sources: Health and potential uses. Phytother Res. 2018 Sep;32(9):1688-1706. doi: 10.1002/ptr.6109.

[545] Antibacterial and antifungal activities of thymol: A brief review of the literature. Food Chem. 2016 Nov 1;210:402-14. doi: 10.1016/j.foodchem.2016.04.111.

[546] Effects of Thyme Extract Oils (from Thymus vulgaris, Thymus zygis, and Thymus hyemalis) on Cytokine Production and Gene Expression of oxLDL-Stimulated THP-1-Macrophages. J Obes. 2012; 2012: 104706. doi: 10.1155/2012/104706.

[547] The Therapeutic Potential of Rosemary (Rosmarinus officinalis) Diterpenes for Alzheimer's Disease. Evid Based Complement Alternat Med. 2016; 2016: 2680409. doi: 10.1155/2016/2680409.

[548] Carnosic acid protects against 6-hydroxydopamine-induced neurotoxicity in in vivo and in vitro model of Parkinson's disease: involvement of antioxidative enzymes induction. Chem Biol Interact. 2015 Jan 5;225:40-6. doi: 10.1016/j.cbi.2014.11.011.

[549] A randomised double-blind placebo-controlled pilot trial of a combined extract of sage, rosemary and melissa, traditional herbal medicines, on the enhancement of memory in normal healthy subjects, including influence of age. Phytomedicine. 2018 Jan 15;39:42-48. doi: 10.1016/j.phymed.2017.08.015.

[550] The role of rosemary extract in degeneration of hippocampal neurons induced by kainic acid in the rat: A behavioral and histochemical approach. J Integr Neurosci. 2018;17(1):31-43. doi: 10.3233/JIN-170035.

[551] Anti-stress and neuronal cell differentiation induction effects of Rosmarinus officinalis L. essential oil. BMC Complement Altern Med. 2017 Dec 22;17(1):549. doi: 10.1186/s12906-017-2060-1.

[552] Effects of Rosmarinus officinalis L. on memory performance, anxiety, depression, and sleep quality in university students: A randomized clinical trial. Complement Ther Clin Pract. 2018 Feb;30:24-28. doi: 10.1016/j.ctcp.2017.11.004.

[553] Rosemary (Rosmarinus officinalis) as a potential therapeutic plant in metabolic syndrome: a review. Arch Pharmacol. 2016 Sep;389(9):931-49. doi: 10.1007/s00210-016-1256-0.

[554] Anethum graveolens: An Indian traditional medicinal herb and spice. Pharmacogn Rev. 2010 Jul-Dec; 4(8): 179–184. doi: 10.4103/0973-7847.70915.

[555] The effect of 12 weeks Anethum graveolens (dill) on metabolic markers in patients with metabolic syndrome; a randomized double blind controlled trial.

Daru. 2012; 20(1): 47. doi: 10.1186/2008-2231-20-47.

[556] Anethum graveolens and hyperlipidemia: A randomized clinical trial. J Res Med Sci. 2014 Aug;19(8):758-61. PMID: 25422662.

[557] Lipid Lowering Effects of Hydroalcoholic Extract of Anethum graveolens L. and Dill Tablet in High Cholesterol Fed Hamsters. Cholesterol. 2015;2015:958560. doi: 10.1155/2015/958560.

[558] The Role of Anethum graveolens L. (Dill) in the Management of Diabetes. J Trop Med. 2016;2016:1098916. DOI: 10.1155/2016/1098916.

[559] Aqueous Extract of Anethum Graveolens L. has Potential Antioxidant and Antiglycation Effects. Iran J Med Sci. 2016 Jul;41(4):328-33. PMID: 27365555.

[560] Suppressive impact of anethum graveolens consumption on biochemical risk factors of atherosclerosis in hypercholesterolemic rabbits. Int J Prev Med. 2013 Aug;4(8):889-95. PMID: 24049614.

[561] Unravelling the genome of Holy basil: an "incomparable" "elixir of life" of traditional Indian medicine. BMC Genomics. 2015; 16(1): 413. doi: 10.1186/s12864-015-1640-z.

[562] Tulsi - Ocimum sanctum: A herb for all reasons. J Ayurveda Integr Med. 2014 Oct-Dec; 5(4): 251–259. doi: 10.4103/0975-9476.146554.

[563] Essential oil from Ocimum basilicum (Omani Basil): a desert crop. Nat Prod Commun. 2011 Oct;6(10):1487-90. PMID: 22164790.

[564] Hypoglycemic effect of basil (Ocimum basilicum) aqueous extract is mediated through inhibition of α-glucosidase and α-amylase activities: an in vitro study. Toxicol Ind Health. 2012 Feb;28(1):42-50. doi: 10.1177/0748233711403193.

[565] Phytochemical Profile and Evaluation of the Biological Activities of Essential Oils Derived from the Greek Aromatic Plant Species Ocimum basilicum, Mentha spicata, Pimpinella anisum and Fortunella margarita. Molecules. 2016 Aug 16;21(8). pii: E1069. doi: 10.3390/molecules21081069.

[566] Effectiveness of antimicrobial formulations for acne based on orange (Citrus sinensis) and sweet basil (Ocimum basilicum L) essential oils. Biomedica. 2012 Jan-Mar;32(1):125-33. doi: 10.1590/S0120-41572012000100014.

[567] Black pepper and health claims: a comprehensive treatise. Crit Rev Food Sci Nutr. 2013;53(9):875-86. doi: 10.1080/10408398.2011.571799.

[568] Black pepper and its pungent principle-piperine: a review of diverse physiological effects. Crit Rev Food Sci Nutr. 2007;47(8):735-48. DOI: 10.1080/10408390601062054.

[569] Neuroprotective and Anti-Aging Potentials of Essential Oils from Aromatic and Medicinal Plants. Front Aging Neurosci. 2017; 9: 168. doi: 10.3389/fnagi.2017.00168.

[570] Piper nigrum and piperine: an update. Phytother Res. 2013 Aug;27(8):1121-30. doi: 10.1002/ptr.4972.

[571] The effects of black pepper on the intestinal absorption and hepatic

metabolism of drugs. Expert Opin Drug Metab Toxicol. 2011 Jun;7(6):721-9. doi: 10.1517/17425255.2011.570332.

[572] Piperine enhances carbohydrate/fat metabolism in skeletal muscle during acute exercise in mice. Nutr Metab (Lond). 2017; 14: 43. doi: 10.1186/s12986-017-0194-2.

[573] Piperine, an active principle from Piper nigrum, modulates hormonal and apo lipoprotein profiles in hyperlipidemic rats. J Basic Clin Physiol Pharmacol. 2006;17(2):71-86. PMID: 16910313.

[574] Curcumin and Piperine Supplementation and Recovery Following Exercise Induced Muscle Damage: A Randomized Controlled Trial. J Sports Sci Med. 2017 Mar; 16(1): 147–153. PMID: 28344463.

[575] Cinnamon: Mystic powers of a minute ingredient. Pharmacognosy Res. 2015 Jun; 7(Suppl 1): S1–S6. doi: 10.4103/0974-8490.157990.

[576] Cinnamon use in type 2 diabetes: an updated systematic review and meta-analysis. Ann Fam Med. 2013 Sep-Oct;11(5):452-9. doi: 10.1370/afm.1517.

[577] The effects of cinnamon supplementation on blood lipid concentrations: A systematic review and meta-analysis. J Clin Lipidol. 2017 Nov - Dec;11(6):1393-1406. doi: 10.1016/j.jacl.2017.08.004.

[578] Potential benefits of cinnamon in type 2 diabetes. Am J Lifestyle Med. 2012;7:23–6. doi.org/10.1177/1559827612462960.

[579] Dietary cinnamon supplementation and changes in systolic blood pressure in subjects with type 2 diabetes. J Med Food. 2011 Dec;14(12):1505-10. doi: 10.1089/jmf.2010.0300.

[580] Protective effects of cinnamon bark extract against ischemia-reperfusion injury and arrhythmias in rat. Phytother Res. 2018 Jun 19. doi: 10.1002/ptr.6127.

[581] Effect of cinnamon (Cinnamomum verum) bark essential oil on the halitosis-associated bacterium Solobacterium moorei and in vitro cytotoxicity. Arch Oral Biol. 2017 Nov;83:97-104. doi: 10.1016/j.archoralbio.2017.07.005.

[582] Meat consumption, Cooking Practices, Meat Mutagens and Risk of Prostate Cancer. Nutr Cancer. 2011; 63(4): 525–537. doi: 10.1080/01635581.2011.539311.

[583] Heterocyclic amines: Mutagens/carcinogens produced during cooking of meat and fish. Cancer Sci. 2004 Apr;95(4):290-9. PMID: 15072585.

[584] Plant extracts, spices, and essential oils inactivate Escherichia coli O157:H7 and reduce formation of potentially carcinogenic heterocyclic amines in cooked beef patties. J Agric Food Chem. 2012 Apr 11;60(14):3792-9. doi: 10.1021/jf204062p.

[585] Inhibition of heterocyclic amine formation in beef patties by ethanolic extracts of rosemary. J Food Sci. 2010 Mar;75(2):T40-7. doi: 10.1111/j.1750-3841.2009.01491.x.

[586] Inhibitory effect of fruit extracts on the formation of heterocyclic amines. J Agric Food Chem. 2007 Dec 12;55(25):10359-65. PMID: 18004801.

[587] Fruits and vegetables protect against the genotoxicity of heterocyclic aromatic amines activated by human xenobiotic-metabolizing enzymes expressed in immortal mammalian cells. Mutat Res. 2010 Dec 21;703(2):90-8. doi: 10.1016/j.mrgentox.2010.08.007.

[588] Inhibitory activity of Asian spices on heterocyclic amines formation in cooked beef patties. J Food Sci. 2011 Oct;76(8):T174-80. doi: 10.1111/j.1750-3841.2011.02338.x.

[589] Heterocyclic aromatic amines in deep fried lamb meat: The influence of spices marination and sensory quality. J Food Sci Technol. 2016 Mar; 53(3): 1411–1417. doi: 10.1007/s13197-015-2137-0.

[590] Inhibitory effect of mixture herbs/spices on formation of heterocyclic amines and mutagenic activity of grilled beef. Food Addit Contam Part A Chem Anal Control Expo Risk Assess. 2018 Aug 23:1-17. doi: 10.1080/19440049.2018.1488085.

Last But Not Least

♪CHAPTER 16

My Wish for You

I sincerely hope that this book and the mini guide, a separate pared-down version of this book, have opened your eyes. It is extremely important that we all continue what Gary Young started almost three decades ago. His message to the world is just so important for our health and wellbeing.

We will soon be in big trouble. As a medical doctor, it is my mission and duty to educate the public about the dangers affecting our health rather than just bandaging the symptoms.

If we do not stop destroying our bodies and damaging the environment, we will see a continuation in the fall of fertility rates. All these pollutants are basically endocrine disruptors and are causing havoc on both male and female fertility. And because of the epigenetic changes mentioned several times in this book, we will influence the health and diseases of generations to come.

The Bible in Exodus 34:7 says that God "visits the iniquity of the fathers upon the children and the children's children to the third and fourth generation." By applying the field of epigenetics, modern science might now have an explanation for this statement.

I do not think there is something like the "Perfect Life." Life is life because of its joys and sorrows. However, I am convinced that we can make a significant difference for ourselves, our families, our pets, all animals, and the environment.

Being a Young Living member also means being part of a large international family. That family should rise together to make a difference. This book provides an easy way to get started in that direction, with the scientific references to prove it. Please share this information and this opportunity with everyone you care about. Together, we **will** make a difference!

-Doctor Oli

Olivier Wenker, MD, DEAA, ABAARM, MBA, Fellow in Integrative Cancer Medicine, Fellow in Metabolic and Nutritional Medicine

What's coming next from Doctor Oli?

I have been using Cannabidiol, aka CBD, with and without essential oils for several years. I have experienced CBD's potential power firsthand, especially when combined with the right essential oils. Over the years I created a variety of CBD and EO blends to support healthy organ systems and overall wellness. It is time to share those with you.

I realize how much confusion surrounds the topic of CBD. While some know exactly what CBD is and where it comes from, in general, many people are utterly uninformed. My goal is to shed some light on the Cannabis plant and the difference between CBD and THC, to discuss the current status of confusion among the lawmakers, and to recommend exactly what to take and at what doses.

It is time to dive into the details of CBD and why it goes hand-in-hand with essential oils. Did you know that CBD has poor bioavailability when taken orally? Luckily there are several tricks, like adding the correct essential oils, to boost the effects of CBD. And because CBD and certain essential oils have similar chemical constituents, they can be easily combined.

Sign up for my emails at DoctorOli.com to be the first to know when this book releases, and become your own expert in combining the world of hemp with the world of essential oils.

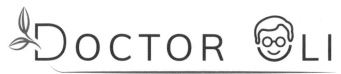

DoctorOli.com

Postcards, Mini Guides, Books, Bundles and More!

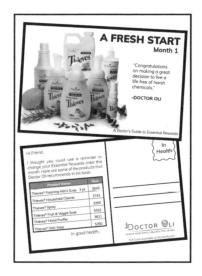

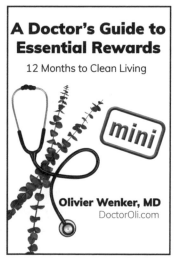

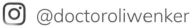

Connect with Doctor Oli

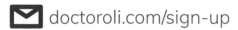

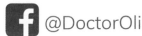 doctoroli.com/sign-up

@doctoroliwenker

@DoctorOli

PRAISE FOR
A Doctor's Guide to Essential Rewards

This is an excellent resource!! I love this book for guiding individuals month-by-month towards a non-toxic lifestyle! Every chapter is scientifically referenced supporting the value behind the Young Living products. This a must-have book as it gives valid explanation for each choice toward a healthier lifestyle.

As the founder of the Healing Home Movement twenty years ago, my heart jumped with excitement to have a book like this to back up our message. From our gut to the great outdoors, we have a month by month teaching guide supported by scientific resources. This serves as a third-party validation for those sharing our message! I have known Olivier Wenker, MD as my physician and as a personal friend. I have trusted his guidance through my own health journey and have respected his counsel.

So having his explanation and his endorsement is a game changer in sharing the impact Young Living can have on our daily lives. His integrity comes from a true desire to help others, and he always gives above and beyond expectation in his professional and personal life. He is respected by thousands around the world as an educator. With that said, I know you will appreciate this impactful book and how it will add back-up credibility to your message!

Connie Marie McDanel, Royal Crown Diamond, Healing Home Movement, Co-Author of Aroma Home & Aroma Clean

Doctor Oli has had my heart since the first moment I met him—not because he is spectacularly smart (which he is), or has a resume longer than a dozen doctors (which he does), or because he is a gifted speaker and writer and researcher that I deeply respect, or because he was Gary's personal medical consultant and had the ear of the man that founded this company, or even because he loves his two kids and his wife and serves them more than anything else in the world. He has my heart because he is honorable, humble, and has every quality that Gary Young would look for in his closest friends. Oli dreams like Gary. I believe he is one of the few men left on this earth that truly encapsulates the spirit of Gary Young in every single way.

Why should you read this book—or anything that Oli writes? Because he has decades in the medical field and sees the world of oils through a professional lens. Because he is also a gifted writer who can articulate why it's so critical for you to have oils in your home and USE them every day, and he can explain it in a way you've never heard before- not as an aromatherapist, but as a medical doctor and scientist with a knack for making complex concepts simple. Because he was the trusted confidant, friend, and global traveler to and with Gary Young, and has decades of his knowledge stored away in his head—projects they have worked on together and whispered behind walls. It is knowledge we'll lose forever if it's not written down. You should read this book because Oli has the tenacity and fight to train you to be the protector of your home, family, and body. And the whole world will be better with this man's wisdom. He has forever changed my life. And now he is about to change yours.

If you act on what you read, it will dramatically change the way you look at oils in your home. Every bottle will have new purpose, significance, and meaning. But most importantly, read this book and pass the knowledge of Gary through Oli to those you meet. If you do that, you will have a hand in getting Young Living Essential Oils in every home of the world.

And that is why we do what we do. Not to sell, but to train. Without training, there is no understanding or knowledge of how to care for ourselves. Your health is your greatest gift! Without it, there is no thriving family and no way to pursue your calling and purpose. Oli has spent his life teaching people preventative maintenance and self-care. This book is his precious gift to us. You can read it and put it on a shelf, or you can change the world one bottle at a time. It's time for us to pick up where Gary left off.

Sarah Harnisch, Mom of Five, Lover of Jesus, Young Living Diamond and International Speaker, Radio Network News Anchor in Chicago and New York, Amazon Best-Selling Author of the Gameplan Series (1.5 million sold!)

Doctor Oli's new book A Doctor's Guide to Essential Rewards *packs an incredible punch if you're looking for a health do-over. He's one of the most well-respected physicians who teaches integrated lifestyle changes over pushing pills. This book will help you understand the why, what, and how when it comes to making a permanent healthful shift in your choices and habits.* A Doctor's Guide to Essential Rewards *is full of relevant research to back up his healthy shift suggestions and it will help his readers to have zero excuses when it comes to choosing health!*

Jen O'Sullivan, Author of 6 Best Sellers. Creator of The EO Bar and Live Well Apps.